"Anger goes up, Fear goes down - Emotions and the hidden link"

Ancient healing principles and treatments that can change your life

by

Cairo P Rocha

This book is a work of non-fiction. Names of people and places have been changed to protect their privacy.

First published by AuthorHouse 06/24/04

ISBN: 1-4184-6044-3 (e-book)
ISBN: 1-4184-2807-8 (Paperback)

Printed in the United States of America
Bloomington, IN

This book is printed on acid free paper.

Acknowledgments

I would like to express my gratitude to:
Linda Osborn, a multi-talented friend, who patiently reviewed this manuscript.
Cheryl Lam for kindly proofreading this material.
Raquel Rocha, my niece, who posed for the stretching sketches.
My patients and students, who have taught me so much.
My families - in Brazil and the Bahamas - for their constant support.
Cara Christie, my wife, whose tireless support and encouragement have made this book a reality.

To

Cara, my wife,
my best friend and the
radiant energy behind
everything I do.

TABLE OF CONTENTS

PART ONE

Emotions and their powerful effect on us

Understanding Chinese medicine

What causes diseases?

Emotions and health - The Hidden Link

Fear, Anger, Worry, Sadness, Joy, Anxiety, Shock, Hatred, Guilt, Craving and Love

Depression

Self-sabotage

Introduction

From the very beginning of my practice as a Japanese-Chinese medicine therapist, I have come across a variety of cases where emotions were the underlying cause, whether obvious or hidden. Looking back over the years, I can even pinpoint the moment where everything started.

It happened in 1990, in Brasilia, Brazil. I had just opened my first clinic and was excited at the possibility of putting into practice everything I had learned in my eight years of study abroad. Anna, a polite and soft-spoken lady, came to see me because she was suffering from an excruciating pain in her right leg, just above the knee. She had tried all the conventional therapeutic methods with no success. From the Chinese medicine standpoint, that meant energy stagnation. Thus, with that idea in mind, I started needling some acupuncture points that the case recommended. However, the moment I inserted a tiny needle in the painful spot, the lady started to cry, first gently, then convulsively. I was shocked at Anna's reaction and feared that I had badly hurt her. Because she was one of my first patients, I thought that my career as an acupuncturist was not going to be a long one. Immediately I proceeded to remove the needles and saw her going away still crying.

On the following morning, to my surprise, there she was again in my waiting room. Luckily, she was not crying anymore - actually she had a smile on her face! She told me that the night before, the very night she had had the acupuncture session, she had a vivid dream. She dreamed that she was on a big black ship and that she was being whipped on the leg, exactly on the same painful spot. The dream (or nightmare) stirred up intense emotions, such as fear, anger and hopelessness. Amazingly, when she woke up in the morning, the pain was completely gone. There was no trace of it!

I was astounded by the whole episode. Anna's case was a major revelation to me, for up until then, I had regarded acupuncture as a very effective therapeutic tool for treating physiological disorders. All of a sudden I was facing a new dimension that would, from that moment onwards, cause a significant shift in my understanding of the human being's limitless dimensions.

Anna's experience could be understood as a "trapped" emotion in her muscle-skeletal system. From the therapist's point-of-view it is irrelevant whether the causing factor could be found in past-life circumstances or if the dream was just a metaphor resulting from the imbalance brought about by the pain. In my opinion, the most important aspect of the case is that an unresolved emotional issue, which in Chinese medicine could be translated by "stagnated energy", was manifesting itself through a physical pain. Moreover, by stimulating the painful spot, the energy had been released. Interestingly, after that whole episode Anna said that she felt as if a "big weight" had been lifted from her body and that fear, a constant companion, no longer bothered her.

Three main conclusions can be drawn from the case:

1) An emotion has energy of its own which can manifest itself physically - one can't deny pain;
2) Emotions can be accessed and dealt with by any therapy that contemplates the energy concept.
3) Once the stagnation is removed, the causing factor (emotion) disappears and, consequently, the physical discomfort ceases.

The majority of holistic therapy practitioners are familiar with the fact that a trauma, whether physical or emotional, leaves scars or sequels in our biomagnetic field, which can be interpreted as a disturbance in the flow of energy throughout our body, according to the ancient Chinese. From the therapist's point of view, it is not so relevant "when" the trauma occurred; the most important factor is that the body still "remembers" it and reacts whenever a similar situation comes about. It is like an allergic reaction.

With allergies our body's defenses overreact against a substance it *considers* to be harmful to its integrity. What follows then is a chain reaction that can be very uncomfortable and even life-threatening. Likewise, having experienced a trauma charged with emotion in the past, every time we come across a similar situation, our energy network gets "fuzzy", like a TV that is not properly tuned. The incident

3

involving a dog described on page 32 is a good example. The alarm goes off and the same emotion felt in the past is triggered together with physiological symptoms.

David Elman, a renowned hypnotherapist, believes that allergies are closely related to repressed emotions. In his opinion, every case of hay fever represents a "crying syndrome". The eyes tear and get red as from weeping, the nose runs, and the throat gets dry and raspy. Frequently, there is gasping for breath. All these signs appear when a person cries excessively. Hypnoanalysis reveals again and again that victims of hay fever and many other respiratory illnesses have undergone traumatic experiences that caused prolonged crying. Consciously, these people have stemmed back the tears, but at a level below conscious awareness the tears persist. The crying apparently affects a change in sensitivity to allergens, and the allergic reactions develop in the crying syndrome of hay fever. Tears are one of nature's best relief mechanisms and should not be repressed.

It is not necessary to be a therapist to understand the whole picture. We are all aware of the effects that emotions have on us, sometimes in a very subtle way but other times, in quite a tangible form. We don't simply experience an emotion - we "feel" it. The following situations are just a few examples of some of our physical reactions to emotional states:

- Just by thinking of a lemon or tamarind pulp → *reaction*: the mouth gets watery in a matter of seconds
- At the beginning of a romance, you are told "I love you" → *reaction*: shaking legs, pounding heart and a sensation in the stomach
- When facing a great fear → *reaction*: tightening of the muscles, pale face, cold hands and urinary incontinence
- Experiencing an outburst of anger → *reaction*: clenching of the jaws, tightening of the fists, a bitter taste in the mouth, a strong headache or loss of consciousness
- Feeling sad → *reaction*: tightening sensation in the chest, sensation of blockage of the throat, tears
- Worry → *reaction*: uneasy sensation in the stomach, cold and sweaty hands
- Guilt → *reaction*: shallow breathing and heavy sensation in the limbs
- Depression → *reaction*: total lack of energy, the mind feels stagnated and the muscles lethargic
- Emotional upset → *reaction*: constipation or diarrhea, dysfunction of the heart's pulsation.

The above situations illustrate the close connection between mind/emotion and the physical body. Emotions have energy that can manifest in a variety of ways, either by triggering the release of hormones in our blood or, as we are about to see, by affecting the flow of *CHI* (vital energy), a cornerstone concept of Chinese medicine.

The motivation-force behind the idea of writing this material was to share my own experience in dealing with emotional issues with the general public. Throughout the following pages the reader will be able to have a better understanding of the link *mind-body-emotion;* to detect early signs of disease and to have a special close-up of the internal mechanism of the emotions. It is my utmost desire that the information presented in this book contributes to making a positive difference in your life.

Chapter I

Emotions and their powerful effect on us

As a therapist, I have come across many cases of physical disharmonies untreatable by our mainstream medicine, where the cause could be traced back to early childhood traumatic experiences. A good number of them are caused by those unwritten rules, like "Men don't cry" - for crying is a sign of weakness; "Flowers are for women" – men are not supposed to like flowers; "Children are to be seen, not heard" – children are expected to keep their thoughts to themselves; just to name a few. Of course those unwritten rules are predominant in certain cultures and were stronger in our parents' generation.

Stammering, for instance, although vaguely considered a pathological disorder, is normally caused by an emotional trauma at an early age. In the book "Hypnotherapy", Dave Elman explains that stammering or stuttering has its root in a situation where **the child is not allowed to cry**. Hypnoanalysis, a therapeutic technique that can locate the cause of many emotional traumas through hypnosis, has demonstrated that in innumerable cases.

I have an interesting case that can perfectly illustrate the power of a repressed emotion on a physical level. Mary, a thirty-five-year old woman with a severe case of Bell's Palsy or facial paralysis, came to me for acupuncture treatment. Normally, this problem responds well to acupuncture, especially in the early stages.

The treatment was carried out for over six months with positive results. However, because there were strong emotional issues behind the physical problem,

I decided to integrate hypnotherapy into the acupuncture treatment. The interesting aspect about her problem is that she had come down with the paralysis when her husband went ahead with an important project for the family without her consent.

Through hypnosis I assisted her regression back to childhood, when she could picture herself clearly at a table with the family. She is the only daughter of a large family. Although she has a loving mother, her father has always been very authoritarian and, in her view, only gives special attention to her brothers (she considers herself as being just an "appendix"). She feels that she has never had a **say**, much less when she was a child.

With this emotional pattern going on for so long, it was not difficult for me to realize that because she was not able to express herself, her body "created" the paralysis - her mouth got twisted. As we know, the mouth is the ultimate element responsible for speech. Moreover, according to Chinese medicine, speech is related to the Heart* (the Heart governs the mind); therefore we can picture the following development:

Emotional trauma→Heart + speech blocked→paralysis

With all this information in mind, I decided to have her confront and solve the problem in the environment that felt particularly difficult to her: at mealtimes. The suggestion was that she had the unique opportunity to express her feelings freely; everyone else was frozen and all ears. She began by saying everything she wanted to say to everyone, but when I suggested she tell her father how much she cared about him, despite his attitude towards her, **she felt her mouth twisting and moving to the side, exactly the same way the paralysis affected her.** To make a long story short, she was encouraged to open her heart to the whole family, to forgive everyone, to forgive herself and to be free. After that, her physical and emotional improvement was noticeable in many ways.

Again, one has to acknowledge that the above mentioned rules were stronger in our parents' generation and nowadays the old ways are being systematically questioned. However, it is very important that we therapists, teachers and parents, are aware of the damage caused by repressed emotions. As we shall see in the following lines, emotion is energy, and in Physics it is well known that energy can be controlled until it finds a loophole to manifest itself in a powerful and uncontrolled way. What is the connection between mind and body? Where is the link? We shall explore this subject in detail in the following pages.

The main idea is that once we know the close relationship between a particular organ and a specific emotion, as well as the effects of the emotion in our bodies, we will be able to detect the origin of disturbances considered beyond our mainstream medicine's reach. I could be bold enough to say that all diseases, especially those that develop slowly in our body, have, without exception, their roots in a powerful emotional issue trapped in our energetic field. Consequently, as all the gardeners know, the only way to get rid of a stubborn weed is by removing the roots. Hopefully the information presented here will bring some light to the roots of problems that currently affect people in modern society, both in the physical and emotional realms.

* Incidentally, the use of capitals when writing organs' names is intentional. The idea here is to differentiate the organs as Western anatomy describes them (small letters) and the Chinese medicine approach (capital). Therefore, whenever we come across an organ's name written in capitals it means *the energetic aspect of the organ.*

Chapter II

Understanding Chinese Medicine

Since the very beginning of my practice I have always been fascinated with acupuncture's range of action - it can treat a variety of conditions such as pain, disharmonies of the internal organs, addictions and emotional problems, just to name a few.

Situations involving traumas, behaviour, relationships, family disharmony and similar issues are important aspects of my work. Even though I am not trained in traditional psychology, I have found that when one immerses oneself in Chinese medicine, the emotional aspect of the problem (whether obvious or hidden) is of great importance when it comes to choosing the proper line of treatment. Incidentally, modern psychology has been around for 150 years or so, but most of the issues dealt with by Western psychologists nowadays were known to the Chinese more than 2000 years ago.

The decision to write this book came from the desire to share the ancient Chinese approach to emotions and how they affect our body. Up until now this knowledge was reserved mostly for Chinese medicine scholars and therapists, which makes it difficult for the general public to have access to this important and useful information. In the following pages the reader will have an overview of Chinese medicine and consequently, be able to understand the powerful link of **mind-body-emotion**. In order to learn the foundations of ancient Chinese medicine, one needs to grasp the notion of three main concepts: *Chi, Yin/Yang and the Five Elements.*

Chi

CHI or Qi can be roughly translated as *vital energy.* It is both life energy permeating the whole being, physical, mental and spiritual, and a cosmic energy identifiable with the Hindu *prana*, the Greek *pneuma* and the Hebrew *hua*; it is the basic force of the universe. Whenever a Western scholar tries to translate the Chinese language he/she always faces the same challenge: the characters represent not only a sound, but also an image or a concept. However, the idea of Chi meaning the energy that is behind every movement or phenomenon of the Universe is pretty close to the way the Chinese themselves understand it. Chi is the energy behind the birth of a star, a comet's trajectory, our body's functions and the flapping of a butterfly's wings. Natan Sivin, in "Chinese Alchemy" writes:

> " On one level it names the air we breathe, the subtle material breath of life. In cosmology it is used for a terrestrial effluence, through which the planets move. In chemistry it can refer to an aroma, to fumes, to smoke, or to the activity of a reagent. In medicine the homeostatic force within the body is Chi, so is any pathological agent which disturbs the balance, so, for that matter, is abdominal gas...In translating, therefore, one must choose between carrying over the larger concept of the particular sense...When an author specifies that the alchemical vessel be tightly luted so that the Chi of the volatile ingredients may not escape, one naturally chooses "vapours" as the equivalent which makes his intention clearest, but one loses the implication unless it is kept in mind that Chi means activity too. "

Throughout the centuries the Chinese observed Nature's harmonious and continuous movement. The ever-changing cycles like night and day, the four seasons, the stages of life: birth, maturity and death; all these were carefully and patiently observed by the ancient Orientals. They also understood that as part of Nature, we human beings are subject to the same movement. Every phenomenon of the Universe, everything that moves needs energy and the energy is called Chi. Chi is life; the absence of Chi is death.

Lillian Too, in her book "Applied Pa-Kua and Lo Shu Feng Shui", draws an elegant concept of Chi:

> "To the Chinese, CHI is the mysterious inner energy, which gives strength and soul to mankind. CHI is created when a monk sits in deep meditation and expertly controls his breathing; each time a Kung Fu

master delivers a well-aimed blow; when the artist calligrapher makes an exquisite brushstroke. In each of these activities a special kind of inner vitality accompanies the movement to create a unique power, a life force that chaperons the breathing, the blow, and the brushstroke, making each of these actions distinctive and superior. These are manifestations of human CHI."

In Japan the idea of Chi (or Ki in Japanese) is so imbedded in the local culture that many martial arts, therapies and daily words contain it, for instance:

- Aikido: a Japanese martial art developed by M. Ueshida and can be translated as **Ai** meaning to Unite or Combine; **Ki** is the energy, and **Do** means the Way or Path - "The Way of United Energy".

- Tai-**Ki**oku-Ken (Tai-**Chi**-Chuan): the "Great Ultimate Energy" (**Ki** or **Chi**) uses rhythmic movements and breath control to bring Yin-*Yang* forces into harmony.

- **Ki**koo (**Qi**gong or **Chi**kun): the ancient Chinese healing art that combines gentle movements with deep breathing, self-massage and meditation.

- Reiki: can be translated as "Universal Energy" - **Rei** means Universal; **Ki** is the Energy. It is an art rediscovered in the 1800s by Mikao Usui and consists of channeling healing energy through the hands.

- Genki: health (or healthy Ki); it is a very common form of greeting: *Genki desu ka?*, meaning How are you? (or literally: *Are you healthy?*)

- Byo**ki**: disease (or diseased Ki)

- **Ki** no yowai: faint, fainthearted (weak Ki)

- **Ki** no hayai: hasty, quick, hot-tempered (fast Ki)

- Ten**ki**: lightning (or heaven's Ki) - lightning (fire), father and earthquake

- **Den**ki: electricity (or earth's Ki)

- **Ki**sha: steam-powered train

- **Ki**teki: steam whistle

- **Ki**sen: steamboat

The image of Chi flowing through our body within channels is undoubtedly the cornerstone of Chinese medicine. William Ten Rhyne, a XVII century Dutch surgeon was, perhaps, the first Westerner to write about the action and effect of Chi in the body. While stationed in Nagasaki, Japan, as a member of the Dutch East Indian Company, he witnessed therapeutic methods unknown to him being applied with amazing results. In his book "De Acupunctura", which is considered the first detailed Western treatise on acupuncture, Ten Rhyne describes, for instance, the insertion of very thin needles into specific points of the body for therapeutic purposes. He explains that the aim of this kind of treatment was to promote the flow of energy, which he calls "Spiritus". To him is attributed the creation of words like "acupuncture" and "meridians" (or channels).

Chinese medicine arrived in Japan around the VII century AD. From the beginning of that century Japan started sending missions to study in China on a regular basis, and at the same time, Buddhism and its philosophy applied to medicine also arrived. Although therapies like acupuncture and herbalism originated in China, their practice spread to other Asian countries like Japan, Korea and Vietnam and, over the centuries, they have changed and adapted to local customs. From Japan, Portuguese Jesuit priests brought the first accounts of these fascinating medicines that even now, centuries later, challenge the Western mind.

The idea of cultivating and mastering Chi (energy) for martial arts and healing purposes is widespread in Asian countries. Qigong is one of them. As we have seen above, Qigong or Chikun is an ancient Chinese healing art that combines gentle movements with deep breathing, self-massage and meditation. It is known to improve the circulation, strengthen both the immune system and the internal organs, clear the mind and reduce stress. I have found its practice to be particularly beneficial when dealing with emotion-related problems.

There are health care facilities in China that apply Qigong as the main therapy for terminal diseases, like cancer. The Shanghai Hospital is one of them. Michael Tse, a renowned Qigong practitioner writes:

> *" It (Qigong) is widely used as a treatment for cancer in China, helping the patient fight the problem by building more Chi through exercise and relaxation. When you practise Qigong, your body becomes stronger...The Chi from practice is like a dam, it is holding back the cancer cells, preventing them from growing. It is also fighting to overcome them as well. Your body is relying on the Chi rather than strong medicine or operations".*

One of the Chinese medicine practitioner's first diagnostic steps is the evaluation of the Chi, mainly through body inspection, tongue examination and the palpation of the pulses, a technique that requires experience and skill. Pulse Diagnosis is a refined diagnostic method, whereby the therapist touches both radial arteries (simultaneously or one at a time) proximal to the wrists, in order to assess the condition of the energy flow in each organ, the relationship amongst all of them as well as detecting the presence of any Pathogenic Factor (disease causing agent) in the body.

Interestingly, the use of the pulses as an examination method is said to have originated in ancient China, when the noble ladies were not supposed to expose their bodies for examinations. All the therapist could see was their hands resting on a small pillow isolated from their bodies by curtains. Therefore, the therapists had to develop a fairly reliable diagnostic technique based only on what they could see and touch!

You have probably seen or heard the following situation: someone has a health problem or pain, which leads him/her to go through all kinds of tests and nothing is found. "This must be stress, a psychosomatic problem or a result of depression", to name just a few of the most common mainstream medicine's diagnostics to the above conditions. The patient may not get relief for his/her problem, but at least he/she is given a label! From the Chinese medicine's point of view, the explanation lies in the fact that the disharmony is still on the energy level and, therefore, can only be detected and dealt with by a therapy system that involves the concept of Chi.

It is well known by Chinese medicine practitioners that before the disease manifests in our body, there is a disruption in the energy flow quite often caused by unbalanced emotions. As we are going to see later on, a long-standing emotional problem can eventually affect the organ to which it is related. Thus, a present overlooked emotional issue could well become a physical problem in the future.

Another way to visualize the importance of Chi flowing in our body is by comparing it to a system of irrigation - canals through which water irrigates a plantation. If there is enough water flowing, the plants will be healthy and strong; if there is any blockage preventing water from nurturing the plants, they will eventually wither and die. In such cases, we need to find out where the blockages are and remove them. Roughly speaking, that is what acupuncture does.

The channels or meridians are pathways in which the Chi circulates. The twelve regular meridians plus two extra ones are distributed symmetrically at the left and right sides, and the midline of our body. Each one of them contains a certain number of points, also called acupoints, where acupuncture, acupressure or other stimulation techniques are applied. During the course of an acupuncture treatment, the therapist normally stimulates a combination of points with the purpose of harmonizing the flow of Chi, whether the problem is physical or emotional.

One of the most frequently asked questions is "How can an Oriental medicine practitioner foresee a disease that may only manifest in the future?" Well, with the concept of Chi in mind, one can project the actual picture into the future. In other words, if the present pattern of energy imbalance continues it will eventually change into a physical disease. Also, the emotional aspect involved in the picture can play a very important role, as we will be able to see later on.

In order to better understand the concept of Chi, it is also important to take into account that the energy that flows throughout our body is basically the combination of two sources: the Pre-natal CHI and Post-natal CHI.

Pre-Natal Chi

The Pre-natal CHI or Inherited CHI is the Chi that is transmitted by the parents to the child exactly at the moment of conception. This type of Chi will assist the development of the fetus and the early childhood cycles, and is stored in the Kidneys as the "essence" that nurtures all the body's structures.

The Chinese place special emphasis on the parents' health, as being very important to the quality of the child's vitality. This will certainly determine how well the child will face and deal with health imbalances throughout life. The Orientals even suggest ways of preparing for the sexual act aimed at the conception of a new being. It is important that the parents be in good health, not be exhausted after a long day's work, and be without the effect of alcohol or drugs (being drunk can significantly damage the energy transferred to the child), etc.

Let's consider that you are known to be a conservative type of person. You don't like wearing bright colours (especially red), shorts or hats of any kind. One day you are invited to a party in the countryside. It is a beautiful sunny day and you decide to walk around a nearby pond. All of a sudden, you step on a stone, lose your balance and fall into the water. You are now soaked, wet and dirty. The hostess takes pity on you and suggests you take a shower and to put on dry clothes. The problem is that she has got only a change of green shorts and a red shirt. Well, between the idea of having nothing to wear or accepting her offer, you hesitantly take the clothes. After a while you are comfortably enjoying the party, when somebody decides to take a picture of all the guests in front of the house. However, precisely at the moment when the photographer presses the button, somebody quickly puts a hat on your head. So, your image frozen for posterity is of a person wearing shorts, a red shirt and a hat, regardless of your actual likes and dislikes. That is exactly the image of the "moment" of conception, when the father's Chi blends with the mother's and is transferred to a new being.

It would be quite unfortunate, however, if you had to count only on a Chi inherited from your parents. Luckily, there is also another source: the Post-Natal Chi.

Post-Natal Chi

As the name suggests, this is the Chi that we acquire after birth through the food we eat and the air we breathe. So, if there isn't much we can do about the Inherited Chi, it is possible to control the quality of the Chi we bring into our bodies. It is, therefore, very important to pay attention to our diet and the air we breathe. Smoking is considerably detrimental to our health - it poisons our vital energy.

It is not by chance or coincidence that in all Oriental practices, like Yoga, Qigong (Chi Kun), Tai Chi Chuan, just to name a few, breathing plays a very important part. The air we breathe is charged with energy, which makes Chi move all over our body, promote the elimination of toxins, nurture the brain and induce relaxation. Research has proven that during times of stress, anxiety and worrying, the brain waves move very fast; these are called *beta waves*. Through breathing they can significantly slow down, similar to the waves measured during meditation (*alfa waves*), or even slower (*theta waves*), like those observed during deep sleep. The Orientals say: "When you are overwhelmed and stressed out about a problem or a decision to make, stop everything, close your eyes, be still like a tree and take a few deep breaths. You may be able to see the problem from a different perspective and to find a solution afterwards."

As for food, the Chinese have always considered food as a prime medicine. A well balanced diet should be enough to maintain our health and to promote healing.

What is the first thing that comes to your mind when you think about Chinese food? This is a question I frequently ask my students. The answers are normally chopsticks, spring rolls, sweet and sour dishes, etc. In fact, going to a Chinese restaurant is quite an experience as our senses are exposed to all kinds of flavours, colours and aromas. However, since the Chinese are considered to be a very practical and down-to-earth people, there must be a very good reason for all this variety. There is one indeed.

According to the Chinese tradition, each flavour has an effect on a particular organ; for instance, **sweet** flavour relates to Spleen and Stomach; **spicy** - Lungs and Large Intestine; **salty** - Kidneys and Bladder; **sour** - Liver and Gall Bladder; and **bitter** - Heart and Small Intestine. Ideally, in one meal there should be all five flavours in order to nurture the corresponding organs. Another important consideration is that too much of a good thing can be harmful for instance, if the Liver is considered to be in "excess" (hyperfunction), eating sour or acidic food can create more disharmony. It would be equivalent to pumping more air into a balloon that is about to burst! It is therefore important to investigate the cause of a problem, before deciding what kind of food is suitable to the case.

Throughout China there is a special kind of restaurant called "Yo-San". This kind of restaurant, also known as "medicinal restaurant", applies the Chinese therapeutic approach to food. At the entrance, there is a Chinese Medicine practitioner who evaluates the customer's health condition. After some consideration, he writes a prescription indicating what kind of food is suitable for that particular person. The customer then presents the paper to the waiter, who hands it to the chef. Thus, the meal prepared for him/her will follow the therapist's recommendations as to what kind of ingredients it should contain.

The above example shows the unique Chinese approach to food. Food is energy and the lack of or limited variety of it can generate disharmony. Therefore, it is easy to understand why the use of strict diets does not resonate with Chinese medicine. Again, if each flavour nurtures a particular organ and food is the main source of the Post-Natal Chi, we should be always aware of the quality and the variety of it throughout our lives.

The best way to understand Pre-Natal Chi and Post-Natal Chi is to see the former as a Savings Account that you want to save for old age, and the latter as a Current Account where you can deposit and withdraw as necessary.

An acupuncturist friend of mine recently dealt with a case that illustrates the above paragraph. A twenty-year-old man was brought to him in a very poor condition. He was extremely debilitated and couldn't stand on his own - he had to be carried by his elder brothers to the clinic. Upon careful examination, my friend noticed that the individual was suffering from severe Chi deficiency. However, how could that be happening to such a young man?

After a long talk with his patient, the therapist learned that he had a very active sexual life, smoked like a chimney and didn't care much about eating. Then, it all made sense: the Post-natal Chi was not being properly replenished and the body was drawing heavily on the reserves (Pre-natal Chi), which were probably weak. The treatment: the young man was to spend a long time in the countryside, abstain from smoking and from sex for a long period of time and to have plenty of nurturing and energetic foods. Months later the young man came to his clinic for another evaluation and, to my friend's amazement, he had become a strong and healthy man.

Circulating Chi means life, health and harmony. Blocked Chi means stagnation, disease and death. This concept was well known to the Chinese thousands of years ago and with this concept in mind, they endeavoured to develop therapeutic methods to promote the flow of Chi. Acupuncture, herbs, diet, massage, martial arts, and breathing exercises are some of the techniques created to harmonize the circulation of Chi and to promote health.

Incidentally, the word *alchemy* means to the majority of us a science practiced in medieval times, whose main goal was to find ways of transforming any metal into gold. Chinese alchemy, being more concerned with longevity and immortality than making gold, was naturally involved in finding the Elixir of Immortality and ways of promoting solid health. That is why all the emperors were always surrounded by good and famous therapists. However, the story goes that, in an attempt to attain immortality, many noblemen shortened their lives by drinking poisonous potions.

The Polarities Yin & Yang

If I were to sum up Chinese medicine in a few words, I could say that it is a therapeutic system based primarily on the interplay of YIN and YANG. Yin and Yang are qualities or different polarities, which complement each other and are the common denominators of all phenomena of the Universe.

This concept was first registered about 700 BC, in the "I CHING", "The Book of Changes", where Yin and Yang are represented by broken and unbroken lines respectively. Nature's cycles inspired the Chinese's extraordinary capacity of observation. As we give wings to our imagination, we can picture peasants observing the constant alternation of night and day, the changing seasons, and the birth, growth and death of all living beings on the face of the Earth. In trying to understand and to interpret Nature's ways, the ancient Chinese created a whole philosophy, which (over the centuries) has been strongly influencing their lives, values, culture and, of course, the medicine.

The idea behind Yin and Yang is very simple, yet profound with many ramifications. They are tangible concepts but at the same time ethereal, like a ball of cotton candy, for instance.

The Chinese characters that represent Yin and Yang originate from the following image:

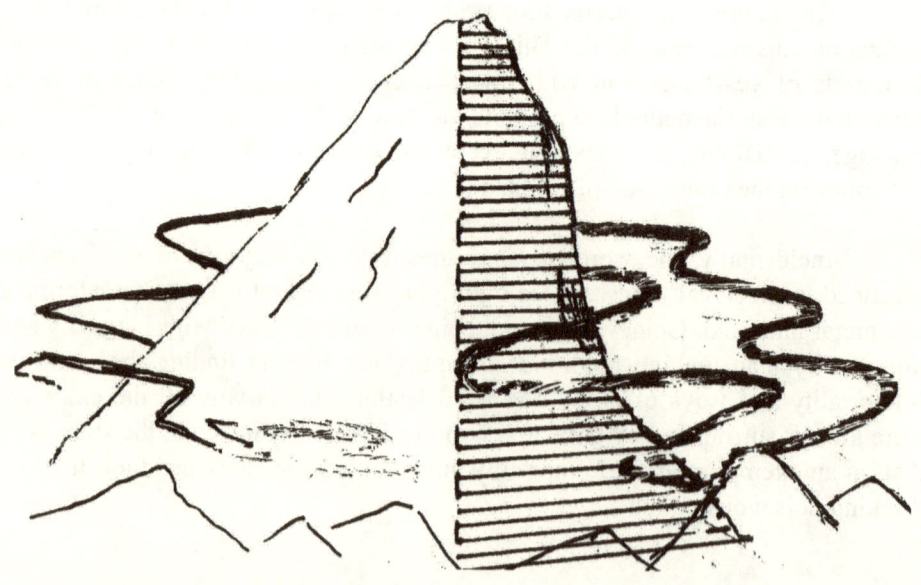

YANG : **The sunny side of the mountain** YIN : **The shady side of the mountain**

Based on the above picture, the following ideas unfold:

Yang	Yin
Light	Darkness
Day	Night
Sun	Moon
Heaven	Earth
Heat	Cold
Fire	Water
Activity	Rest
Severe	Gentle
Hard	Soft
Round	Flat
Time	Space
Immaterial	Material
Generates energy	Generates form
Energy	Matter
Expansion	Contraction
Above	Below
Outward	Inward
Masculine	Feminine
Dried	Wet
Excitement	Inhibition
Fast	Slow
Transformation, change	Conservation, storage

In terms of human body and medicine we have:

Yang	Yin
Hard areas of the body	Soft areas
Back	Front
Upper parts	Lower parts
Skin, surface	Internal organs
Hot sensation	Cold sensation
Acute disease	Chronic disease
Fast onset	Slow onset
Quick changes	Slow progression
Restless, insomnia	Sleepiness, apathy
Body and extremities hot	Body and extremities cold
Loud voice, talkative	Low voice, quiet
Strong breathing	Superficial and weak
Thirst	No thirst
Red face	Pale face
Prefers cold drinks	Prefers hot drinks
Dark and scanty urine	Clear and profuse urine
Constipation	Soft stools or diarrhea

The concept of two polarities that complement each other is fascinating, because one can easily observe them at play in Nature. Life, as we know it, cannot exist in total darkness or in total light; meaning there must be an alternation between night and day. In daily clinical practice the understanding of Yin and Yang manifestation in our bodies is a very important element for diagnosis. For instance:

- A patient expressing himself/herself through wide gestures, loud voice and showing signs of restlessness indicates Yang condition; while a person moving slowly, speaking in a low voice and showing signs of shyness indicates Yin condition.

- The habit of sleeping on the stomach, curled up or with layers of blankets regardless of the temperature, show signs of Yin condition; whereas the habit of sleeping outstretched, lying on the back or with no cover regardless of the temperature, indicates Yang condition.

- The preference for cold food or drinks, regardless of the exterior temperature indicates Yang internal condition; on the other hand, a preference for hot food and drink shows signs of Yin condition.

- A disease that manifests through signs of fever, redness of the skin, thirst and agitation is considered to be a Yang condition; whereas a health disturbance manifesting through paleness, chilliness, sleepiness and absence of thirst is regarded as being a Yin condition.

The emotions can also be classified into Yin and Yang. Fear, Guilt and Worry are considered to be Yin; whereas Anger and Joy are Yang.

The Theory of the Five Elements

Whenever two or more acupuncturists are engaged in conversation, one might possibly hear expressions like: Earth is depleted, Fire is in excess, Water is not controlling Fire, Metal insults Wood, etc. For somebody who is not familiar with Chinese Medicine terminology, the expressions above sound rather strange. However, the Theory of the Five Elements together with the concepts of Chi and the polarity Yin/Yang are the main foundations of Chinese medicine.

According to Giovanni Maciocia, in his book "Foundations of Chinese Medicine", the theory of the Five Elements and its application to medicine mark the beginning of what one might call "scientific" medicine and a departure from Shamanism. Until then, disease was believed to be a punishment inflicted on mortals by angry gods. From that stage onwards the healers no longer looked for a supernatural cause of disease; they now observed Nature and, with a combination of inductive and deductive methods, they would look for patterns and apply them in the interpretation of disease.

The interaction amongst the Five Elements (Wood, Fire, Earth, Metal and Water) is considered to be the core of all phenomena of the Universe, according to the ancient Chinese. With the understanding that the microcosm reflects the macrocosm, we have the Five Elements represented in our bodies: Wood is represented by Liver and Gall Bladder; Fire is represented by Heart and Small Intestine; Earth is represented by Spleen and Stomach; Metal by Lung and Large Intestine; and Water by Kidney and Bladder.

The best way to understand the use of the Five Elements in diagnosis and treatment is through their interrelationship. The most important ones are two:

1 - "Mother and Child Relationship" (Generating Sequence) - In this relationship each element generates or nurtures the other, in the following sequence:

- Wood generates Fire: wood feeds fire; therefore **Wood is Fire's mother**.

- Fire creates Earth: earth is generated by fire (magma), thus **Fire is Earth's mother**.

- Metal is created in the Earth; therefore **Earth is Metal's mother**.

- Metal transforms into liquid, when melting; therefore **Metal is Water's mother**.

- Water nurtures Wood; therefore **Water is Wood's mother**.

In clinical practice, whenever one element is considered to be weak or deficient the "mother" is normally "supplemented" or reinforced, since a well-fed mother is more capable of feeding her child. A practical example: in the case of weakened Lung, its also important to strengthen Spleen, because Lung belongs to Metal and Earth (Spleen) generates (nurtures) Metal.

2 - "Husband and Wife Relationship" (Controlling Sequence) - In this sequence, each element controls another, in the following order:

- **Wood controls Earth**: a tree breaks open the soil with its roots.

- **Earth controls Water**: earth encloses, dams water.

- **Water controls Fire**: water extinguishes fire.

- **Fire controls Metal**: fire melts metal.

- **Metal controls Wood**: metal cuts/saws wood

A good example of the control relationship: when dealing with Liver problems, it is wise to check the Lung and Spleen condition, because Metal *controls* Wood and Earth *is controlled by* Wood.

I would like to give you an idea of how the diagnosis is made by applying the Five Elements Theory. Somebody comes to the clinic complaining of the tendency to catch colds easily. That can trigger the following reasoning:

1. Tendency to catch colds = weak Lung energy = Metal Element deficient
2. Who controls Metal? = Fire. Who is controlled by Metal? = Wood
3. When Metal is deficient (weak) it is right to expect that Fire is exercising its control too strongly over Metal.
4. Now, with Metal deficient, Wood must be too strong because Metal is too weak to control anything.
5. Thus, what we have here is the following equation:

deficient Metal = excess Fire + excess Wood
or
deficient Lung = excess Heart + excess Liver

Let's suppose that we have a situation, where the main characters are a dog, a cat and a mouse. As we know, the dog chases the cat and the cat chases the mouse. Now, what happens if the cat is frail? The dog will overpower the poor cat and the mouse will be free to eat all the cheese in the house. The best solution here is to make sure that both the dog and the mouse are under control, until the cat recovers its strength.

The above reasoning can be applied to our example. The Lung is the cat, the Heart is the dog and the Liver is the mouse. Normally a therapist would choose an approach that would draw the Liver and Heart excess energy and that nurtures and supports the Lung (either by energizing the Lung itself or the Spleen, the mother). The amazing aspect of this approach is that despite its simplicity, the Theory of The Five Elements is alive, and for centuries has been challenging science with its disconcerting effectiveness.

The following table shows the sets of physiological relationships between the Five Elements and body and emotions:

THE FIVE ELEMENTS

WOOD	FIRE	EARTH	METAL	WATER
Liver/ Gall Bladder	Heart/ Small Intestine	Spleen/ Stomach	Lung/ Large Intestine	Kidney/ Bladder
Eyes/ sight	tongue/ speech	mouth/ taste	Nose/ smell	Ears/ hearing
Tendons	blood vessels	muscles	Skin and hair	Bones
Anger	Joy	Worry	Sadness	Fear
Tears	Sweat	Saliva	Mucus	Urine
Sour	Bitter	Sweet	Pungent	Salty
Green	Red	Yellow	White	Black
Wind	Heat	Dampness	Dryness	Cold

Chapter III

What Causes Disease?

The ancient Chinese were aware of a variety of ways of promoting health through methods that harmonize the flow of energy. They also knew the factors that cause blockage or stagnation of Chi. The so-called *pathogenic factors* or disease-causing agents can be of internal or external origin. The external factors are the environment, weather, accidents, radiation, poisons, etc; whereas emotions are considered to be internal disease causing agents.

The exposure to climatic variations should not be automatically considered a Chi blocking factor. We all know that nature has its cycles and under normal circumstances, the weather offers no threat provided we take reasonable precautions, like wearing warm clothes in Winter, impermeable garments on rainy days, wearing light clothes and drinking plenty of liquids in the Summer, etc. Also our body has the means to adjust itself; for instance in cold weather our muscles and the pores contract, whereas in the summer our muscles expand and there is more perspiration. However, when our metabolic and immune systems are weak or out of balance, we become vulnerable to exterior conditions. In Chinese medicine, the climatic factors that can block the flow of Chi and can, therefore, create disease are: Wind, Cold, Dampness, Summer-Heat, Dryness and Fire. As we discussed above in the theory of the Five Elements, certain organs are vulnerable to a climatic element. **Heart and Small Intestine** are vulnerable to **heat**; **Liver and Gall Bladder** are vulnerable to **wind**; **Spleen and Stomach** are vulnerable to **dampness**; **Lung and Large Intestine** are vulnerable to **dryness**; and **Kidney and Bladder** are vulnerable to **cold**.

We can mention a few examples: Brasilia during winter, tends to be very dry and, therefore, cases of lung-related disorders are very common; in Japan, during cold days, the Japanese used to wrap a warm piece of cloth around their waists to protect the kidneys; in places that are damp like the Amazon region or cities on the coast, people tend to suffer from spleen (digestive) disorders, like diarrhea, low metabolism, tendency to accumulate fluids; on windy days individuals prone to liver disorders, tend to experience an increase in headache attacks.

Other pathogenic factors are:

- **weak constitution**: as we have seen above, the parents' health at the time of the conception, plays an important role in the physical and energetic constitution of the individual. Also the mother's poor health and bad habits, like smoking or intoxication with drugs, alcohol, etc, and emotional "turbulence" during pregnancy can leave the unborn child with physical and energetic sequels.

- **over-exertion**: an imbalance between activity or work (whether physical or mental) and proper rest can cause disease. Over-exertion weakens the body and doesn't allow Chi to recover. An old Chinese text says:

*"...excessive lying down injures the Lungs; excessive sitting (*and thinking - intellectual work*) injure the Spleen; excessive standing injures the Kidneys; excessive exercise injures the Liver"*. On the other hand, inactivity and sedentary life can result in stagnation of Chi.

- **excessive sexual activity**: traditionally the Chinese consider excessive sexual activity (meaning: ejaculation for men and orgasm for women) as being cause of disease, for it tends to weaken the Kidneys. However, it is important to say that it is difficult to determine what is normal for somebody or what is excess. Ideally the sexual activity should be determined by one's age, physical condition and health. Giovanni Maciocia, in his book "The Foundations of Chinese Medicine", quotes the book "Classic of the Simple Girl" from Sui Dynasty (581-618 AD) on the ideal frequency of ejaculation for man according to age:

- every 4 days for a 20-year-old; every 8 days for a 30- year-old; every 6 days for a 40-year-old; every 21 days for a 50-year-old and every 30 days for a 60-year-old.

- irregular diet: as mentioned before, diet plays an important role in the quality of Chi circulating in our body. Malnutrition is, of course, the root of many diseases and is present not only in poor countries, but in rich and industrialized ones as well. Food deficiency can result in malnutrition as much as excessive and irregular diet. Strict and rigid diets can considerably jeopardize our health, since our body follows nature's movements and cycles - we change, we evolve. The Chinese main guidelines on the subject are: "Moderation and common sense".

- accidents and trauma: these can cause local stagnation of Chi and blood. A good example of that are certain types of headaches - the ones that only manifest in the same spot are normally a result of an old injury in that area. Moreover, scars resulting from surgery or injury, depending on their location and condition, can block the flow of Chi and can, therefore, create health problems.

Undoubtedly, there are certainly many other pathogenic factors, which we are exposed to and that can cause disease. However, the most powerful one is the effect of an uncontrolled and constant presence of a particular emotion or emotions, which is the main subject of this book that will be discussed in detail.

Chapter IV

Emotions and Health - The Hidden Link

We are all aware of the array of emotions present in our daily lives. Some of them manifest themselves occasionally, while others are more frequent and have become aspects of our personality. Certain emotions are so close to us that they feel like part of our skin - we don't even notice their presence and effects in our relationship with people and in our surrounding environment. In the following pages, I am going to demonstrate how emotions affect our body. What exactly happens inside us when we experience emotions? How do our internal organs deal with the variety of them?

Before showing the energetic side of the picture, it is important to acknowledge that modern science has acquired considerable knowledge of human physiology, pathology and psychology in the last decades. The concept of Psychosomatic Disorders, where emotional states are believed to generate or bring about certain physical problems is considered to be a big leap towards understanding mind-body relationship. It is understood now, for instance, that a long-standing depression can cause cardiovascular and immune system disorders. We now know, for example, that in our brain - a wonderful machine that spends about 20% of all the energy used by the body - there are more connections amongst the brain cells than stars in the Milky Way! Also, scientists have discovered that when we face emotionally stressful situations, our brain releases substances that help us cope with the challenge by defusing the "energetic upsurge", promoting a restful night's sleep, relieving pain and producing pleasure. They are neurotransmitters called Serotonin, Noradrenalin and Dopamine/Endorphin, respectively. People prone to emotional disorders such as anxiety and phobias, and who are predisposed to overstress are believed to have low rates of those chemicals.

It is well known that human beings have never experienced such a high degree of emotional "turbulence" as seen nowadays. We leave the twentieth century with the idea that never in humankind's history has so much been accomplished in such a relatively short period of time. On the other hand, with all our basic material needs satisfied, the emotional issues have never been so strongly present in people's daily lives. Having said that, how does mainstream medicine deal with emotion-related disorders? Well, despite all the astonishing modern knowledge acquired in the schools, hospitals and clinics, when it comes to mind-emotion related problems, the treatments aim primarily at "controlling" the disorders, not curing them. The therapy of choice is the administration of potent drugs that can produce fast results by mimicking the body's own chemical system, but how about the side effects? Is it expected that the individual will spend the rest of his/her life taking drugs? Unfortunately, it seems that the brilliance of our Western medical achievements does not always translate into happiness.

One of the most important and fascinating aspects of Chinese medicine is the holistic approach to the human being. According to the ancient Taoist philosophy, we are more than a physical and tangible body; we are also emotion and spirit. Behind the body's mechanisms there is a blueprint of energy, a concept that Western science finds it difficult to accept. From a Chinese medicine practitioner's point of view, an emotion has the same power to generate disease as a virus. A particular emotional state can "stagnate" our vital energy, "reverse" it's flow, "dissipate" it and "knot" it; strange but accurate terminology that will be explained ahead.

According to Zhuang Zi, one of the greatest Taoist philosophers from the 4th century BC, "We need emotions and feelings because, how could we exist as individuals without them?"

It is important to say that, under normal circumstances, emotions are not causes of disease. Like rivers, emotions are forms of energy that need to flow, to circulate and to express themselves. They are intrinsic parts of us; they are our identity and the manifestation of our humanness. The typical serene image of Buddhist monks totally exempt of emotions does not correspond to reality. They do experience emotions; they are vibrant and jovial, like Soggyal Rimpoche, a famous Tibetan Lama, and also called "The Laughing Tibetan". Serenity does not mean lack of emotions, but the control of them. When someone is serene, he is not disturbed by emotion, or if he is disturbed he is easily able to find his balance again.

It is normal to experience a variety of emotions during the day: anger while driving to work; fear in the dentist's waiting room; worry about a school test; sadness at the news that someone in the family has died; joy at the birth of the first child, etc. It is basically impossible to live and to be part of this world without experiencing emotions, which, provided that they are transitory, have little significance to a Chinese medicine therapist. However, whenever there is a predominance of one or more emotion, they could become pathogenic factors and deserve close attention.

In Chinese medicine, emotions, when considered disease-causing agents, can disturb the flow of Chi (vital energy) and blood circulation, and damage the internal organs. On the other hand, the condition of the organs can directly affect our emotional state. For instance, fear can damage the Kidneys and unhealthy Kidneys can manifest externally through fear, thus creating a vicious circle.

According to ancient Chinese texts: *"Anger injures the Liver; Joy (excessive) injures the Heart; Grief and Sadness injure the Lungs; Worry injures the Spleen; and Fear injures the Kidneys."* This statement is based on the theory of the Five Elements. However, the Chinese also consider pensiveness, shock, hatred and guilt as disease-causing agents as well. As we shall see later on, a certain emotion can affect more that one organ, such as sadness affecting the Lungs and the Heart. As a matter of fact, all the emotions manifest themselves indirectly through the Heart, which is the "Seat of the Mind", according to Chinese medicine. Interestingly, in Chinese, the character representing "Heart" is present in basically all characters related to emotions.

In the following chapter, we will be discussing each individual emotion and the effect it can cause in the organs. The "hidden link" is Chi, the energy connecting the organ to the emotion and the emotion to the organ. It is not tangible and cannot be measured or analyzed under a microscope, but it is powerful and once harmonized, capable of healing any disease.

Chapter V

Fear

Fear, real or imaginary, can weaken the Kidneys. That means whether you are afraid of a mean dog barking at you or you are frightened that there is a Bogeyman under your bed; the effect on your body, or more precisely, on your Kidneys, is the same.

From the Chinese medicine's point of view, *fear makes the Chi descend*. This can be responsible for situations where a state of fear can cause incontinence of urine or diarrhea. Also quite often, a fearful child can develop nocturnal enuresis (bed-wetting) and, in such a case, threats and punishment only aggravate the problem. The Chinese consider that only at seven years of age is the energy of the Kidneys mature; before that children have a certain tendency to suffer from what is called "Kidney-Chi Deficiency". What follows, then, is a chain reaction:

weak kidneys→fear→enuresis→punishment→fear→weak Kidneys→fear

According to Chinese medicine, the Kidneys manifest in the hair, control the bones, nourish the brain, govern hearing, are responsible for reproduction, and control the opening and closing of the two lower orifices: the anus and urethra (and spermatic duct in men). When the Kidney energy is strong and stable, the hair and the bones (and the teeth) will be strong; thinking will be clear and memory sharp; hearing will be normal and the excretion of urine and feces will be regular. However, a strong fear or a constant state of fear can weaken the Kidneys and affect its functions. It is well known that when facing imminent death, a death row prisoner's hair can turn grey overnight.

While practising in Japanese clinics, I remember an interesting case of a lady whose daughter was attacked by a dog while they were walking in the neighbourhood. The injury was insignificant, but later on every time she remembered the scene, she would experience pain coming from the sole of her foot, moving through the inner side of the leg and reaching the lower back. The lady had been through all kinds of exams and drugs to no avail. Finally, she decided to try Chinese medicine and the therapist, after careful examination found out that the pain moved along the *Kidney channel*! So, after working with the Kidney energy and psychotherapy, she reported no more discomfort.

Another important aspect of the Kidneys' function, in Chinese medicine, is the relationship between Water and Fire. The two elements, represented by the Kidneys and the Heart respectively, complement each other in the sense that Water goes up to cool down Fire and Fire goes down to warm Water. In practical terms, whenever Water (Kidneys) is (are) weakened by fear, it can't cool down Fire (Heart) causing anxiety, restlessness and excess perspiration - typical symptoms of a frightened individual.

It is also important to point out that fear itself does not always have a negative quality in our lives. Lack of fear can be responsible for imprudence and unnecessary risks. In a right dosage, fear can allow the person to be vigilant and alert; therefore, this emotion can ultimately be life saving. One can say that normal fear is the reaction one feels when threatened, while abnormal is fear out of all proportion to the scary object or event. Pathological fear, however, is a permanent state of mind that continues long after the fearful event has passed.

In my practice I have been experiencing interesting results by combining Chinese medicine with hypnotherapy for cases of hidden or manifested fears. In both situations it is important to find the cause, defuse the trauma or the "programme" stored in the subconscious mind, and strengthen the Chi of the Kidneys. In other words, both cause and effect should be treated for healing to occur.

A "programme" can be defined as an idea that has been planted in our subconscious mind, and that has a considerable effect on our daily lives. If it is a positive one, it can be an important asset in helping us to deal with all challenges and obstacles; on the other hand, if it is a negative programme, it can prevent us from achieving even the most basic goals in life. In other words, a stone in the shoe! Unfortunately the latter is more common, especially fear-generating ones.

Childhood is the time when we are most vulnerable to external input, whether reasonable or not. Because a child's mind is still immature and doesn't have the "filters" that we adults develop as we grow older, a bad programme can be easily "installed". This is particularly true when we begin to interact with other children at school. Comments like "You have such a big nose", made by an insensitive child, whether true or not, can generate poor self-esteem that might affect the person throughout life. This can be a major cause of unreasonable fears as well.

A hypnotherapist friend of mine once came across a difficult case of fear of an unknown cause. Her patient, a pretty thirty-year-old lady, came to her searching for help to ease her problems. Despite the fact that she apparently had no reason to be unhappy, she was extremely insecure, with a strong fear of rejection and poor self-esteem. The most awkward aspect of her problems was that she "dreaded" those hospital double-moving doors! For some reason, the sight of those doors triggered some strong fear reaction inside her.

One day, under hypnosis, she recalled a very interesting scene of her early childhood. It was more precisely soon after she was born. She was the youngest member of a couple who already had three daughters. When her father went to see her at the maternity room, and as he was pushing the doors (those doors!) he said jokingly, "If it is another girl, I am going to send her back". Somehow the baby registered that comment! All her psychological challenges seemed to have originated then and there. Interestingly, upon realizing that, the fear of hospital doors disappeared as well as many of her emotional problems.

As we have seen before, becoming aware of the circumstances that created the bad programme is already a significant step towards healing. However, from Chinese medicine's point of view, a long-standing state of fear can weaken the Kidneys' energy. It is also important to strengthen the Kidney-Chi in order to achieve the best results.

Body language can be a good indicator of how the emotions affect us and, more precisely, what part or parts of our physical body is/are involved. Fear can trigger the following reactions:

contracted body → reduced blood circulation in the extremities (Chinese
                  medicine: disharmony between Heart and Kidneys)
paleness → same as above
cold limbs → same as above

dry mouth → Kidney, Spleen and Lungs being affected
shakiness → presence of adrenalin in the blood (fight or flight hormone),
released by the adrenal glands (Chinese medicine: Kidney Chi unstable)

Anger

A good image of anger is that of fireworks: they go up and explode in the air. That is exactly how the Chinese describe the energetic picture of anger in our body: *anger makes the Chi rise.*

Anger, from the Chinese perspective, injures the Liver and this emotion, if constantly present in somebody's life, can cause syndromes like "the rising of the Liver Yang", or "Liver depression with Chi stagnation". For those who are not familiar with Chinese medical terminology, the first syndrome can manifest through the following symptoms: throbbing headaches, ringing ears, dizziness, vomiting, convulsions and even stroke. The second syndrome can be headaches, constipation, myomas, menstrual problems, depression, etc.

Again as stated before, when anger is out of control or if it has been part of someone's life for a long time, can become a disease-causing agent. The Liver Chi's main function is to facilitate all movement in the body, like blood and fluid circulation, for instance. This applies to emotions as well. If Liver is depressed with Chi stagnation, there will be energy blockages in many areas of the body, for example: throat - difficulty in swallowing; chest - heaviness in the chest; breasts (women)- tenderness in the breasts prior to menstruation; abdomen - bloated sensation; intestines - constipation, to name a few. There can also be a sensation of life going in "slow motion" or as if "one is driving the car with the hand break on".

It is important to bear in mind that the term *anger* in Chinese can also mean other emotional states, such as resentment, frustration, irritation, animosity or bitterness. If it is not properly channeled it will certainly affect the Liver energetically and physically.

It is also important to consider that the Liver Chi has a tendency to move upwards; anger only intensifies this predisposition. Indeed, when somebody is angry, the face turns red, the eyes sparkle and the person is bound to lose control of his/her actions. "It went to my head!" You never hear somebody saying, "I was so angry that my feet went red." Incidentally, the best acupuncture points to treat

Liver excesses (especially those caused by anger) are in the feet. The idea is to draw the energy downwards.

A good way of certifying the relationship (anger-Liver/Liver-anger) is to place or to hold the hand on the right hand side of the abdomen (at the end of the ribcage) of somebody who is angry; there will be a considerable amount of heat. It is an interesting, yet dangerous experiment!

The Chinese have a saying: "If you are angry with somebody, count up to nine, eighteen, twenty-seven, or even up to thirty-six. At thirty-six, you should be calmer; if not, then you are entitled to punch the person in the face".

The most important energetic aspect of anger is its *up and outward movement.* With this image in mind one can understand the causes and effects of anger in our body.

Beside its damaging effects in the Liver and in the Heart, anger can also be understood as a powerful catalyst. A certain amount of anger or the energy released by it can "stir things up", remove obstruction and also promote necessary physiological reactions in the body. It is like a spice, which when properly added can really improve a meal.

There is a tragic story of a famous Chinese therapist who was called to treat a prince seriously ill due to a blood clot. The therapist decided to provoke the prince in order to make him angry and, as a result of that, the prince vomited the blood clot, which saved his life. However, he got so angry with the therapist that, before his cure, he killed him.

From the therapist's point of view, it is much easier to deal with imbalances where anger is involved, than with low energy emotions like guilt, for instance. Anger, being a powerful emotion with lots of "steam", can be channeled towards the person's own benefit. The energy as raw material is there. In cases where the predominant emotion is low key, it is necessary to stimulate or build the general Chi before anything else can be done. A good example of this is a hot air balloon. It only takes off when there is enough hot air inside it; otherwise it goes nowhere.

Body language: piercing eyes, contracted muscles, clenched fists, flushed face

Worry And Pensiveness

Worry is perhaps one of the most common emotional causes of disease in our society. The fast and dramatic changes in all aspects of life in the past decades have created a climate of such insecurity that, as Giovanni Maciocia points out, "only a handful of Taoist sages are immune to worry."

Preoccupation, a synonym for worrying means to *occupy in advance*. Occupying oneself with a situation that might not even happen is a waste of energy and poses a considerable stress in the body, especially in the digestive area. In Portuguese there is an expression that says it all: S*wallowing frogs!*

Worry knots Chi, according to the Chinese. That means that it causes stagnation of energy in the Spleen, the organ that is energetically responsible for thinking and ideas. It can also affect the Lungs because when one is worried breathing is shallow.

Pensiveness consists of constantly thinking about something, a typical characteristic of an Earth (Spleen/Stomach) type of person. As well as people who worry a lot, there are people whose profession constantly stimulates their intellects, i.e., intellectuals, scientists, accountants, lawyers, writers, etc. These professions can, by causing people to "overthink", lead to problems of the digestive system. The main symptoms are poor appetite, epigastric discomfort, abdominal distension and pain (especially if one worries at mealtimes).

According to Zen-Buddhism philosophy, mealtimes are regarded as being sacred times. Ideally food should be eaten peacefully, in silence (or at least turbulent subjects should be kept away from the conversation), and all devices should be turned off (like TV, radio, telephone, etc).

Speaking of Buddhism, there is an interesting story. Two monks, one senior and one novice, were on their way to a far distant monastery. A pouring rain made them slow down and take refuge under a large tree. When they resumed the journey, they saw a young lady trying to cross the road, but because of her long dress, she couldn't jump over the mud. The senior monk swiftly helped her crossing the road by carrying her in his arms and placing her gently on the other side. She deeply expressed her thankfulness and they proceeded to the monastery. The novice was speechless. He thought, "How could the master do that. He should have known that we are not supposed to touch women!" And so he went ruminating on this thought until late at night, when finally, they arrived at the monastery. Then, not being able to restrain himself any longer, he questioned the senior about the episode. The master smiled and said, "Well, I carried the lady from one side of the road to the other, but it seems that you have been carrying her since then."

Some people, however, due to a constitutional disharmony in the internal organs, like Spleen, Lungs or Heart, are prone to worry, even about insignificant incidents in life. Worrying is also called "Mothers' Syndrome" and it is very common to find mothers worrying excessively about their children. I have come across a case, where the lady always insists that whenever the family is travelling on an airplane, that either she or her husband must fly separately with the children in case the aircraft should crash. In such cases, external factors like insecurity only enhance a pre-existing condition. It is important to find out the roots of the problem, decide upon the appropriate treatment, and make sure that Chi flows freely without any restraint.

I once had a patient who was chronically worried. He would worry about not being on time for the appointment, about the size and the number of needles used during the acupuncture treatment, the duration of the session and, of course, he never allowed himself to relax. One day, in the latter stages of the treatment, something unusual happened. While he was lying in a comfortable position, he yawned a couple of times and fell deeply asleep - a major breakthrough!

<u>Body language</u>: contracted body, cold sweat, hands clasped together at stomach level

Sadness

Unfortunately, we have heard many times that after the death of a loved one, a person develops a serious disease and dies. Was it caused by sadness? From the Chinese medicine's point of view, the answer is "yes", indirectly.

According to the Oriental perspective, sadness reduces and stagnates Chi in the chest affecting primarily the Heart and weakening the Lungs. *Lung governs Chi and sadness dissolves Chi.* The Lung is considered to be the "Minister of Foreign Affairs", because amongst its other functions, it controls the skin (moisture and the opening/closing of the pores). Being the most "exterior" organ, it controls the "Defensive Chi", which is believed to be our first line of defense. We can understand this as being our energetic immune system; our magnetic field. Therefore, the constant presence of sadness or melancholy "dissolving" our Defensive Chi would make us vulnerable to all kinds of disease-causing factors. Also, with the constant input, "I don't want to live anymore" into our subconscious minds, It could bring about a life-threatening disease. Many romantic and melancholic poets have died of pneumonia or tuberculosis in the past!

An old Chinese text called *Book of Rites* talks about the importance of mourning rituals after the death of a loved one. Manifestations like crying are considered to be therapeutic, because they release the stagnated Chi in the Lungs, washing away the sadness.

Here is a good example of the function of Lung Chi in relation to our exterior world: try paying attention to your breathing rhythm next time you feel uncomfortable in an environment, like being at a party where you don't know anybody, giving a speech in front of a large audience or being stuck inside an elevator. It will certainly be shallow. The best way to overcome the problem is by breathing deeply and slowly. How about the situation where one has to face danger, like asking the boss for a raise? What is the first thing one does? Take a deep breath; fill up the chest!

In one of my acupuncture classes in Japan, my main teacher stressed the importance of deep breathing when facing anxiety and stressful situations. Many years later, while I was in Capadocia, Turkey, I decided to visit the underground city dug by the Christians in the past in order to hide from the Ottomans. The city was a large complex of narrow tunnels ending in large caves, like ants' nests. The problem is that, once you are inside, you have to wait for the next group of people to descend, because there is not enough space inside the tunnels. So, there I was somewhere deep down there and listening to the tour guide's explanations. All of a sudden, a thought came to my mind: "What if I wanted to leave? I couldn't do that now…". Immediately, I started perspiring, breathing very shallowly and anxiety took over. Luckily, at that very moment, I remembered my teacher's words and started breathing very slowly and deeply. In a matter of seconds, everything went back to normal. I carried on following my group; nobody noticed anything. That was a major lesson for me.

Another way of understanding the Lung's exterior-interior relationship is by looking into how we relate to other people around us, especially within the family. Whenever there is lack of emotional nurturing, attention or care, imaginary or real, the Lung-Chi becomes stuck, oppressed and incapable of circulating properly. As a result, the individual is prone to Lung related disorders. Being the organ most exposed to exterior circumstances the Lung is prone to be affected by disease causing agents, like wind, cold, dryness and also emotions.

I have two interesting cases that can illustrate the above. The first one was a seven-year-old boy suffering from bronchitis. His father was then a diplomatic attaché and was most of the time away from home traveling or attending meetings, or going to receptions etc. The child was the youngest of four boys and was very close to his mother. In the course of the treatment he was showing significant signs of improvement, not only in terms of health but also at school. However, every time his mother had to accompany the husband in his duties, the crisis of bronchitis got considerably worse and he showed signs of sadness.

Aware of the situation, I talked to his mother about the problem, and we decided that she would do her best to assure him that she would be absent for just a short while and that she should show him signs of special care and affection. Given the circumstances, I decided to incorporate flower essences into the treatment. Flower Essences, as most therapists know, are a very effective form of treating emotional related problems, as we will see in a future chapter. The boy was fine when he left Brasilia and I was told that he is now a happy and strong teenager.

The second case was a middle-aged lady from Norway. We were attending a workshop in Findhorn, Scotland. One day she called me to her room asking me if I could help her, since she couldn't breathe due to an asthma crisis. Upon quickly evaluating the problem, I chose to use moxibustion, an old Oriental technique that consists of applying heat to points or areas of the skin for therapeutic purposes. Since her response to the treatment was very good, I decided to carry on with it on a regular basis. She was doing fine until her daughter called to find out how she was doing. The asthma crisis returned as strong as it had been in the beginning of the treatment.

Given the circumstances, I decided to inquire her about her life, family relationships, childhood, etc. She told me that she had a large family (she had seven siblings) and her mother had never paid her special attention, *unless she was sick*. Having heard that I understood the picture or, at least, I got a good clue of what was going on. In order to attract attention, she had *created* a health problem: asthma. Let's remember that we are talking about a Lung-related disturbance. Therefore, now as an adult her conscious mind wanted to get rid of the problem but her unconscious mind needed it. We had here a tug of war! The best therapy for situations like that is hypnotherapy together with a holistic health care that takes into account body, mind and emotions.

Body language: sunken chest, round shoulders, bent head, shallow breathing

Joy

The reader might find it strange that joy is classified as disease-causing factor. Indeed, joy as a reflex of contentment and happiness is a desired state of mind and is very beneficial to our health. Only when it comes to excessive joy or too much "excitement" can it cause disease. ***Joy slows Chi down and injures the Heart***.

The following story illustrates this point. A long time ago, in ancient China, a young man was promoted to a high-ranking post in the court. One day, as he was walking in the palace gardens, the Emperor's physician, who had been observing him carefully, told him:

"Unfortunately, I have bad news for you. Someone in your family has died and you should go home at once."

The poor man turned pale at the news and made immediate arrangements to travel. However, when he finally got home he realized that nothing had happened, everything was normal. Very relieved and disappointed at the doctor, he returned to the court and asked him why he had done that. The physician calmly explained that the young man was showing an "excess of joy", which could be dangerous to his health. Therefore, he had decided to "apply" another emotion (sadness) to counteract it.

It is indeed well known that excessive joy - like winning a fortune in a lottery or the news that your football team has just won a championship for the first time in history - can cause a person to collapse. Also, in the case of a person with a heart condition, sudden good news can cause a heart attack with serious consequences.

I know of a case of a person who was diagnosed as having bone cancer in its terminal stages. With his days numbered, he decided to enjoy life before it was too late. Since his main wish was to get a driver's license, he took intensive driving lessons. He passed the examination and days later he received the news that he had been granted the driver's license. He suffered a heart attack and died on the spot. He died of joy and was luckily spared of a painful death filled with suffering.

An old Chinese medicine text, "Ling Shu", says: *"When the Chi of the Heart is empty, there is sadness. When it is full, one laughs without being able to stop"*. This is another manifestation of excess excitement affecting the Heart.

The Theory of The Five Elements considers laughter and speech as connected to the Fire Element (Heart/Small Intestine). In cases where the person has speech problems, like stammering or talking non-stop, the diagnosis is disharmony (excess of energy) of the Heart. Likewise, excessive or inappropriate laughter also indicates Heart imbalance. A good example of this is people who laugh when they are nervous or (even worse) at funerals.

Body language: expanded muscles, fast breathing and sensation of warmth.

Anxiety

Do you normally live with a sense of impending doom, a generalized sense that things can go wrong even though there is no real reason for that? Do you usually get to the airport three hours in advance, when you are supposed to be there only two hours prior to the departure? On your way to an appointment when you notice that the traffic is getting heavier, do you normally start sighing, sweating, breathing shallowly and fast for fear that you will be awfully late? Do you usually plan your trips far in advance, in a "surgically" detailed manner that allows no space for spontaneity? If these questions sound familiar to you and the answer to them is "yes", chances are that you suffer from anxiety.

The vast majority of people looking for help at a holistic therapist's office have anxiety as the underlying cause of their problems. It can hide insidiously behind a migraine headache, hypertension or be more openly displayed in psychological disturbances, such as panic disorders, phobias in general and even depression.

The inability of coping with stress is perhaps the main cause of anxiety. This is usually a constitutional or inherited disorder that can be exacerbated by life's challenges upon which one has no control. It is in fact a blend of worry and fear and can also originate from traumatic experiences.

Anxiety stagnates the flow of Chi in the chest affecting primarily the Lungs.

Generally speaking, in Chinese medicine energy stagnation means Liver Chi stagnation regardless of its location. Anxiety is normally accompanied by a variety of symptoms, but sighing a lot, gasping for breath or the sensation that "breathing is not complete" are the most common ones.

Since within the energy concept there is no such thing as an isolated problem, other organs are involved, such as the heart (cold hands, palpitations and insomnia), kidneys and bladder (urge to urinate, lower back pain, dryness in the mouth), and digestive areas (nausea, diarrhea, stomach cramps).

All the above symptoms can occur isolated or in combination but they have, nevertheless, a common denominator: Lungs' energetic dysfunction. As we have seen before, during situations involving stress, worry and anxiety, the brainwaves move very fast and the best way of controlling the situation is by consciously breathing deeply and slowly.

Each one of us has a personal "antidote" to counteract anxiety, even though we might not be aware of it. In other words, intuitively we all have our own way to handle stress by walking on the beach, spending some time in the woods, playing an instrument, or, which is unfortunately very common, eating compulsively. Our body's internal wisdom tries its best to attain equilibrium in order to protect its own integrity.

There is one technique that is as simple as it is effective: yawning! Yawning is a very good and natural way of "defusing" anxiety. Have you ever yawned while on a roller coaster? Or while madly kayaking in the rapids? I don't think so, for we only yawn when we are very relaxed! Thus, it is possible to trigger our body's own reaction to counteract the opposite situation. There is even a therapy called "Yawning Therapy" to help pregnant ladies to prepare for delivery by yawning as much as possible, with the purpose of relaxing the mind, the body and, especially the abdomen. The only problem is that yawning is very contagious and whoever is facilitating the therapy can't go very far before starting to yawn as well. Actually, just by talking about it I am yawning continuously as I write these lines!

<u>Body language</u>: contraction of facial muscles, cold hands, shallow breathing and startling eyes.

Shock, Hatred, Guilt, Craving And Love

Shock scatters Chi and affects the Heart and the Kidneys. Shock causes an internal reaction similar to an "earthquake": the energy is dispersed and as a result of this, the person faints. With the Mind out of control, the "essence" of the Kidneys is drawn as an emergency supply to balance the situation, which creates a considerable disharmony involving Heart and the Kidneys.

A sexual trauma is a good example of this. In cases where the woman is sexually abused, for instance, the shock caused by the aggression makes the *energy move (jump) from the lower abdominal area (reproductive organs) to the Heart.* Consequently, there may be symptoms of menstrual disorders, infertility and hardened emotions, like anger, resentment and bitterness.

Hatred affects the Heart and the Liver. Although very similar to anger in a way that it also affects the Liver and the Heart, it differs in its energetic manifestation. Anger is explosive and makes Chi rise, whereas hatred is a "stiff" and a hardened emotion that, when harboured for a long time, slows downs and stagnates Chi. Hatred can be very damaging to the person who cultivates it and one of its main physical manifestations is pain.

In my practice, I have come across many cases of pain and depression, where the underlying cause was found to be a deep-seated hatred. Sometimes people are not aware of it. Quite often, over the years, the subconscious mind covers up a non-resolved emotion, like layers of sand hiding an old ruin, as a way to protect ourselves and an attempt to make things flow. However, like a hot coal under ashes, it will eventually burn. The only way to deal with situations, where a long-standing and hardened emotion affects the physical body is by "unearthing" it and dealing with it through an external or internal action. Analytical hypnosis can be an effective tool when it comes to locating the obstacle, bringing it up to the light and dissolving it. I have found on many occasions that an integration of hypnotherapy with Chinese medicine can be a very good way of dealing with emotional related disharmony.

Jerry Kein, a well-known American hypnotherapist has a very effective therapeutic technique to dissolve anger and hatred. With the patient under hypnosis, he tells the person to vent all the suppressed emotions by punching a large pillow that he (Jerry) holds. The results are impressive; the only setback is that sometimes the patients get carried away and the therapist suffers the consequences. On one occasion, somebody nearly broke his thumb and another, a football player completely destroyed his office - not a single piece of furniture was left intact. This is just to show the explosive power of suppressed emotions.

Guilt affects the Heart and the Kidneys and it causes Chi to stagnate in the chest, and epigastrium or abdomen. A very common emotion in our lives, guilt can be a result of our past actions or omissions. Violations of social and religious rules are the most frequent causes. "I wish I would have done that" or "I wish I wouldn't have said that" are very familiar thoughts and they keep turning in our minds like a broken record. The worst feeling about guilt is the fact that there is nothing we can do to "mend the broken vase" now.

From the therapist's perspective it is much better to deal with strong emotions, like anger, than with low energy ones like guilt. The former is volatile, alive, yet untamed and can be transformed into a useful therapeutic tool; the latter is heavy, slow and requires a considerable effort to deal with.

Oriental wisdom sees things from a different perspective. The present moment is the most important to us; the here and now. By living the present we are molding our past and our future simultaneously. Feelings that keep us stuck in the past and that prevent us from living our present to the fullest can bring about chaos in the future. Indeed, life is but a colourful collection of experiences that make us whole and mature human beings. We carry with us now the best part of all the past experiences, whether good or bad ones. There is no point in wasting energy by keeping a dead and withered flower; the essence and the perfume have been already absorbed by our soul. No battles, no victories; no experiences, no wisdom!

Craving affects the Heart and scatters Chi. Craving means a constant desire for something that can never be satisfied. The Mind can never be content, settled and peaceful; therefore, the Heart being the seat of Mind cannot relax.

My experience, however, shows that there is also another dimension involved with craving and addiction. Most addictive personalities, who always crave some substance or feel the constant need to "bring" elements into their lives, experienced an emotional void in the past. In most frequent cases, these persons have spent part of their childhood away from the parents (like in a boarding school) and feel the lack of their nurturing presence deep in their soul. The lack of a nurturing (even emotional), base and support can dramatically affect the Earth Element (Spleen/Stomach). I have treated numerous cases of alcohol, tobacco and food additions that confirm this theory, and, only after "filling the void" or tonifying Spleen and Stomach can we achieve long lasting results.

The compulsive eater is a good example of an insatiable desire for food, in order to compensate for something he/she lacks. The most basic and important need for a human being is security. We simply cannot function without minimal levels of security. When facing situations in life that make us feel insecure, our subconscious minds immediately retrieve the sensations of us as babies being nursed in our mother's arms safe and protected. The message that comes is *Food equals Security*. If that is the case, unless we can access that program and erase it, there will be hardly any success in a weight loss treatment.

Love affects the Heart and quickens the Chi. When someone experiences love, the energy (Chi) flows with no restraint especially in the chest, bringing a sensation of lightness and well being. For those who are not familiar with Chinese medicine's diagnostic methods, tongue examination is one of the most popular ones, because it clearly reveals the internal organs' condition.

It is interesting to observe the tongue of somebody in love, for it shows some changes (redness) on the tip of the tongue, which is the area corresponding to the Heart. I was once teaching a practical class at the school's clinic, when, surrounded by students, I approached a patient and ask her to show me her tongue. The patient was a twelve-year-old girl who was accompanied by her mother. After a quick look, I asked her: "Are you in love?" With her face totally flushed, she nodded, much to the mother's surprise. I guess I had involuntarily committed an indiscretion.

Love, as the most sublime of the emotions that a human being can feel, is above all a healing energy. It has the power to transmute and harmonize all emotional imbalances. When the Chinese list love as an energy-destabilizing agent, they mean uncontrolled passion, obsession and jealousy, examples of misdirected love.

A while ago, I heard somebody telling an interesting story. Two Chinese medicine practitioners were on their way to a Tibetan monastery, somewhere in the United States. Despite all their preparation, due to unforeseen circumstances they ended up arriving late at night and everybody there was already asleep. The caretaker, however, took pity on them and offered to prepare a meal. Minutes later she returned with two plates containing rice and fried eggs. When they finished their meal, they wished to know the ingredients of that exquisitely delicious food. She was surprised at their reaction and said that she had not added anything special to the meal, except perhaps lots of love!

Chapter VI

Depression

What you call depression could be just a "running piglet"

I have decided to include a chapter on depression for two important reasons. First, it seems to be the number one emotional problem affecting humankind nowadays. Secondly, depression as seen in ancient Chinese medicine takes a different dimension, as opposed to mainstream medicine's view, in which depression is nothing but a brain chemistry imbalance.

The following lines were written by a patient of mine describing her experience with depression:

It can sneak up as insidiously as a thief in the night, chilling my heart and robbing me of my very self. I feel myself falling...falling...I try desperately to get a grip on myself, to stop this downward spiral into the void, but I am rendered totally helpless to save myself from the agony that awaits me. The terrifying gloom starts to consume me as I reach the bottom of the dreaded abyss. I can see the light at the top but, try as I will, I cannot reach it...Dear God, please, not again!

The blackness begins to swirl in my brain; fear and panic drive out my peace of mind. My normal, well-ordered life, in the twinkling of an eye, is turned into total turmoil. My mind becomes awash with frightening thoughts that whirl round and round, torturing me with their intensity. Molehills become mountains; the simplest decisions become impossible to make. I am sapped of all joy - my usual, ever-ready smile becomes a grimace. I am turned inward, consumed with my own misery, unable to relate to others. It is terrifying because I retain all of my faculties - it would be kinder if I were not so aware. It is almost as though I am outside of myself and another "me" is waiting in the wings, watching with glee my desperate efforts to stop this madness. Truly, if there is hell on earth, I have been there!

Since I left Brazil to study acupuncture in Japan in 1983, I have had the opportunity to live in and travel to many countries. I have spent some time with a Japanese family on a strawberry farm in Hokkaido, Northern Japan; shared a meal with people in the middle of nowhere in Capadocia, Turkey; ridden elephants in Rajastan, India; flown a hot-air balloon over the Valley of the Kings, Egypt; ridden a horse at the foothills of the Himalayas, near Kashmir, Northern India; shared a meal with Sumo wrestlers at their training center, in Tokyo; flown a small aircraft around Mount Everest, from Katmandu, Nepal; conducted a seminar at Bristol Cancer Help Center, England; just to name some of my experiences. During all that time, the most fascinating experience for me as a therapist, has been the opportunity of meeting people, to be somehow part of their lives, and to learn about their lifestyles, dreams, expectations, and emotions.

What I found most fascinating in my travels and experiences, was to realize that no matter in which part of the world I am; no matter how different the customs are; race or religion - the emotions are the same. I have come to know that a Nepalese feels the same array of emotions as a Bahamian, for instance. The only difference is the *way* she/he manifests them. This is very important to me when it comes to understanding people's behavior and the causes and manifestation of diseases.

Another important discovery was that due to climate, geographic location, lifestyles, diet and other factors, there are some health conditions that are typical of a certain country or region. However, there is a problem that respects no boundaries, age or social status: **depression**. It can affect people living in gloomy and cold parts of the world or on bright and sunny Caribbean islands!

Western science considers depression as being the result of an imbalance in the levels of neurotransmitters called "Happy Messengers" (technically known as the Biogenic Amine/Endorphin System). The brain chemicals Serotonin, Noradrenalin and Dopamine are responsible for sleep (body rhythm), energy and pleasure, respectively. The main treatment consists of supplying the brain with the same substance it lacks; in other words, using an external source (synthetic drugs) to supply internal needs. The same procedure is used for insulin dependent diabetics: since the pancreas cannot produce enough insulin to metabolize sugar, they need to have access to external sources for their entire lives.

The body naturally needs to resort to an external supply of substances, like food, water, vitamins and minerals to perform its vital functions. However, despite considerable advances in medicine, the constant supply of external substances (drugs) that the body should be producing on its own cannot be considered the ideal solution. Ideally the body should be able to produce the chemicals and substances necessary for its own needs. One does not need to be an expert in medicine to realize that if areas of the brain are not producing the chemicals to cope with stress, the constant supply of external sources WILL NOT encourage the body's natural mechanism to heal or balance itself.

Again, the Chinese medicine approach to health imbalances, in which not only the physical aspect of the human being is taken into account but also the mind, emotions and spirit, seems to me a well-balanced and sensible one. Another important factor is that we are dealing with a *person*, not a *disease*; therefore, distinct individuals will present similar symptoms, but stemming from different causes.

Not long ago, a sixty-year-old gentleman came to me for a consultation. Although he tried to appear cheerful, his eyes revealed a deep-seated sadness. He carried a heavy label on his shoulders: manic-depressive! (Unfortunately, mainstream medicine is mostly a disease-oriented science and is always ready to attribute labels, which the individual may carry for the rest of his/her life). After a careful examination I told him that from the Chinese medical perspective what was bothering him is called "Running Piglet", a combination of syndromes involving mainly Liver and Stomach-Chi.

In Chinese Medicine, the Liver is responsible for the smooth flow of energy throughout the body and has a profound influence on the emotional state, and conversely, the emotions will influence the Liver's energetic functions. Therefore, if the Liver is functioning well and its energy flows smoothly, the person will be happy and in good spirits. However, long standing repressed emotions like anger, resentment and unfulfilled desires will impair the circulation of Liver energy and cause stagnation. Liver-Chi stagnation is considered to be the main cause of what we Westerners call depression. This syndrome is called *Liver depression with Chi stagnation.*

Again, it is important to say that physiologically speaking, depression can be understood as a result of internal chemical imbalance, as medical science contemplates it. However, it is not quite clear as to what causes the imbalance and as I see it, the Chinese medicine approach is arguably a very sensible one. The blueprint for the condition can only be found in the energy network system, from which health and disease are tangible manifestations of harmonic flow or stagnation respectively.

When somebody comes for treatment for the first time, before deciding which line of therapy is suitable to the case, I have a long and detailed interview with the person. I normally follow a questionnaire specially designed to cover all the aspects of the individual's life, such as present and past health problems, family life, relationships, professional life and emotions. The purpose is not only to know the facts from the person's point of view but also to observe "how" he/she verbalizes them. Voice, gestures and body language are very important tools to detect energetic imbalances.

When it comes to emotions, however, I usually ask, "How do you handle emotions?" Almost always there is a pause. The person is normally taken by surprise and quite often smiles, rolls the eyes upwards and moves in the chair. "Do you tend to keep them inside or do you have your own ways of venting them?" I usually add. "Well… "

That may sound unimportant when the case is clearly diagnosed as migraine headache, for instance. However, based on Chinese medicine principles and on my own experience, this is a highly significant information that could determine the success or failure of the treatment. The most common answer to the question is, "I normally keep them inside." "Has it always been like that?" I inquire further and the answer is quite often, "Yes."

It is amazing the number of people, especially middle-aged ladies in generations from the pre 60's, who have no means of channeling their emotions. With years and years of "poor programming" in a male-oriented society, women have learned to accept the idea that expressing and dealing with their emotions or embracing their inner needs can jeopardize their roles as mothers and wives.

As we have seen before, unfulfilled desires and unexpressed feelings can impair the circulation of Liver's Chi, which according to ancient Chinese medicine is a major cause of what we now call depression. Incidentally, despite the fact that nowadays the challenges are heightened in all areas of our lives and there is a general perception that we live in an increasingly insecure world, not everybody reacts emotionally in the same way. The contingent of men acknowledging feelings of depression is growing, but the large majority are women. They are generally more in tune with their bodies and feelings and, most importantly, the Liver's energy plays a considerable role in female physiology. In Chinese medicine, the Liver is responsible for the uterus and ovaries' functions and menstruation. Therefore, any disturbance in the area suggests Liver imbalance.

More specifically, depression seen by the Chinese consists basically of Liver Chi stagnation in combination with one or more of the following syndromes:

1 - Stagnation of Liver-CHI; suppressing the Spleen

In this syndrome the main symptoms are emotional reticence, emotional depression, crying, suicide desire, rapid emotional changes, poor appetite and loose stools.

As we have seen before in the Five Elements theory, Wood (Liver/GB) controls Earth (Spleen/St); therefore if the energy of the Liver doesn't flow properly it will certainly create problems for the Spleen. Imagine yourself staying in a room with a fireplace activated, the chimney shut off, lots of smoke and windows and door closed. That is the picture portrayed by the Chinese to explain Liver Chi stagnation affecting the Spleen.

In my experience, when Earth (Spleen/St) is energy-deficient the situation gets even worse. The person tends to see no way out and feels powerless to carry on with life. However, when the digestive system improves and the person regains the pleasure of eating, the depression subsides. In other words, if you cannot extinguish the fire or open the chimney, opening the windows could bring some relief.

Barbara, a middle-aged lady and mother of two children, came to see me for digestive problems and lack of energy. She had no appetite, no pleasure in eating and no zest for life. She used to see the world as being "gray". That was a clear case of Spleen Deficiency (lack of appetite and low energy) and Liver Stagnation (no zest for life and seeing the world as being gray).

Since her behavior was pretty much consolidated by old and strict "unwritten rules", I decided to tonify or stimulate the Earth element, i.e., work around the edges. Therefore, with a special diet oriented towards improving her digestive system, herbs and acupuncture, she began to gain strength. Her listless face began to gain colour and her mood changed considerably. One day she told me that she had convinced her husband to go on a cruise - she wanted to explore the world, which in her eyes was no longer "gray".

2 - Stagnation of CHI and Blood

In this syndrome the main symptoms are emotional depression, dejection, crying, foreign body sensation in the throat (like a plum pit), and menstrual disorders (dysmenorrhea, amenorrhea). This is perhaps the most common one and it is usually accompanied by menstrual disorders.

Whenever I notice that there is a sign of energy stagnation, I tend to ask the person, "Do you sigh a lot?" and, "Have you ever had a sensation of a blockage in your throat?" These questions are important to ascertain more precisely where the energy is stagnated. Sighing is a body's natural function to release stagnation in the chest; it feels as if we are trying to catch up with our breathing rhythm. Therefore, if somebody sighs frequently it is a clear sign of feelings or emotions stuck in the chest. As for the sensation of blockage in the throat, that indicates that the energy is stagnated in the vocal area, like unspoken words or non-verbalized feelings.

Painful periods, absence of them or, which is more common, presence of dark blood clots also characterize this syndrome. These are clear signs that the energy is blocked in the lower abdomen. In more severe cases there will be also uterine fibroids and ovarian cysts.

About three years ago, I had a patient referred by a gynecologist friend of mine. Lucia was a young lady suffering from strong depression, irregular periods and PMS. She had tried all kinds of therapy with no substantial results. As it commonly happens, she decided to try acupuncture as a last resort.

One thing I found very interesting: she rarely smiled, normally spoke using short sentences and sighed constantly. She said that she had never been able to convey her thoughts and opinions properly, which was very frustrating. Upon careful evaluation, I realized that Chi was blocked in her throat (unable to speak, to express herself properly) and she had blood stagnation (painful periods). As a treatment I decided to use acupuncture and relaxation techniques, and suggested she sing as much as she could and to do breathing exercises. During the time she was coming for treatment I noticed a considerable improvement in her mood and behavior: she was more talkative, smiled more frequently and ...she had joined a local choir!

3 - Heart and Spleen Deficiency

The main symptoms of this syndrome are chronic depression, vertigo, dizziness, lassitude, weakness and pale complexion, and palpitations. This is very typical of people suffering from a heart condition and /or who have had bypass surgery. The energy is stagnated for lack of "power" to circulate it.

This is a case of not enough blood being built by the body and the heart not being strong enough to pump blood and energy around. One of the most important causes for this condition is the state of the mind. As we have seen before, the Heart is the seat of the mind - meaning the Heart controls the mind and the mind's states affect the Heart.

After a heart attack and bypass surgery, the person feels depressed and contemplates death as being around the corner. We know already that the Fire (Heart/S.Intestine) element generates Earth (Spleen/St). In other words, if the Heart is down we can expect Spleen to be deficient as well, which creates a vicious circle

Depressed Mind→ Deficient Heart→ Deficient Spleen→ lack of energy→ Depressed Mind

I have had many cases like that, especially amongst men, and the best approach is to work with the mind by encouraging the individual to explore the fun side of life. Yes. Laugh at the problem! Many of my sessions are spent telling jokes. Laughing makes the energy flow and removes obstacles especially in the chest area.

It is well known the story of a person who was told by his doctor that his days were numbered, and there was nothing that could be done to save his life. Since he had nothing to lose, he decided to cheer himself up and enjoy the rest of his days. He then rented a good number of comedy videos by the Marx Brothers and checked into a hotel. Encouraged by the positive feeling he was experiencing, he carried on with his "laughing therapy". As a result of that, he recovered his health and strength to his doctor's amazement. Good humour can strongly boost our immune system.

4 - Deficiency of Kidney Yang and Spleen Yang

The symptoms of this syndrome are emotional depression; the person does not feel like speaking; is introverted; refuses to eat, to go out or to see friends; experiences soreness of limbs and knees, impotence, nocturnal emissions, nocturia, and frequent urination. This is a complex case because it has elements of the other three.

The Yang aspect of any organ can be understood as its function, activity and movement. Thus, with Kidney energy (our batteries) and Spleen (transformation of food into blood and energy) being deficient, we have a picture of somebody really "down". This is very common in people who have been battling against a long and debilitating disease, such as cancer. It is like locking oneself up from the world. Having said that, I have known of many cases where the person diagnosed as having a difficult type of cancer understands it as the body's desperate attempt to change, and by consequence develops a remarkable zest for life.

The best therapy for this syndrome is to provide nurturing for the person in all angles of his/her life. I generally recommend a special diet to reinforce the Kidneys and Spleen, herbs for the same purpose and any activity that nurtures the soul. Prayer, meditation and Tai Chi Chuan are some of the best therapies for these cases.

As the reader can see, depression in Chinese medicine doesn't follow one specific pattern - it varies considerably depending on the case. It requires a precise diagnostic and a tailor-designed therapy. The following case is a very interesting one, given its complexity.

One afternoon three years ago, at the end of a lecture I had conducted on "Female Disorders", I was approached by a young lady who wished to make an appointment with me.

Laura, a dark-haired and brown-eyed woman came to me complaining of a long-standing depression. She had a bureaucratic job, which she was not happy with, and had made many frustrated attempts to become an artist, a painter. By looking at her eyes I sensed strong emotions behind them, so I asked her to tell me about herself. With shaky hands and trembling voice, she told me her story.

Her father had died when she was very young, and she was the youngest of four daughters. Her childhood had been normal, without problems, until she had

had an accident. She was 12 years old when, one morning her mother told her to stay home and watch a pot of stew that was being cooked, while she and the other daughters were going shopping.

Later on, while still upset for having to stay home, Laura inadvertently hit the boiling pot, which turned over and spilt the whole contents on her body. Since she was alone, it took a while before a neighbor heard her screaming and took her to the hospital with her abdomen badly burnt. That was the beginning of a series of painful and traumatic plastic surgeries. Ever since that accident, which had left her with large scars, she had been carrying a deep feeling of anger and resentment towards her family for "having left her behind to burn."

Laura's case was anything but routine to me. The emotional wounds were as strong as the physical ones (or even stronger) and since Chinese medicine sees the individual as a whole, I knew I had to address both aspects with equal emphasis. The pattern was clear: depression with long standing harbored resentment pointed at two directions: Liver and Heart. With this in mind, I proceeded to apply the recommended treatment: *free the Liver-Chi; dissolve the hardened emotions; harmonize Heart energy and pacify the mind.* Thus, after six months of treatment, which included acupuncture, Chinese herbs, dietary changes and hypnotherapy, Laura showed a remarkable improvement and emerged as a happy and peaceful person, and she now wants to study Oriental Medicine. Just before I left Brasilia, there was a beautiful *ikebana* (Japanese flower arrangement) on my desk, made by Laura herself, a real proof of her blossoming.

It is normal to question - Why are emotional issues, like depression so much in evidence today? One of the main reasons is that in past generations people were physically busy trying to survive in the fields, fighting against nature's elements with very little technology and comfort. In other words, the *physical* aspect of the human being was more in evidence. Life moved at a relatively slow pace and there was little space for emotional issues. From the energetic point of view, the lower chakras, related to basic survival issues, were the most active ones.

Today, with the fast and astonishing technological advances, our basic needs are met quite simply by pressing a single button. In our modern society we are also being constantly bombarded with a considerable amount of information. Everything is moving fast and we feel as if we are in a never-ending roller coaster. Thus, because we don't necessarily need to use our muscles to survive, and since most of the information that reaches us is cheerless, the upper chakras, the ones related to *emotional* issues are more active then ever.

During all the years I have been involved with acupuncture and related therapies, I have noticed a considerable increase in the number of people who come for treatment, not necessarily for pain-related disorders, but mostly for emotional imbalances. Depression is by far the most common complaint.

For somebody who is not familiar with the syndrome, it seems easy to deal with the disturbance - all the individual has to do is to come out of it! Indeed, it would be an easy issue if it weren't for all the chemical imbalances and energetic underlying causes. Once the disharmony is properly diagnosed, it is possible to treat and cure the condition we call depression. In the following pages, I will discuss some of the therapies that have proven to be effective in treating depression and other emotional disturbances.

Chapter VII

Self-sabotage

I have decided to include self-sabotage in this work because even though it cannot necessarily be considered an emotion *per se*, it is quite often a common denominator in both physical and emotional imbalances.

Whenever a new patient comes for consultation, I normally conduct a detailed interview before choosing the best approach to his/her condition. During this first contact, I have the opportunity to access not only the energetic underlying cause of the problem but also most importantly the person's own evaluation of his/her imbalance. As a rule, I normally pay as much attention to <u>how</u> the patient is speaking as to <u>what</u> is being said. Gestures, body language, eye movements and voice inflections quite often reveal the underlying causes of the problem. Thus, listening carefully is crucial at this point.

When I first began my practice, despite focused attention on the first interview, I often had the feeling that I hadn't gotten the whole picture. Something was missing, and as a result, occasionally I found myself dealing with what I call the "yo-yo syndrome", where a good improvement in the patient's condition was almost systematically followed by an equally strong setback. I remember quite often questioning my therapeutic skills!

According to an ancient Oriental saying, "Light doesn't penetrate a human being's mind in a single flash." As I became more experienced and mature, I realized that I was obviously overlooking an important piece of the puzzle. In the past I tended to rely basically on my own evaluations and on what the person was telling me. That should have been all I needed to get a clear picture of the condition, but it wasn't. There was still a hidden element: **self-sabotage!**

Self-sabotage behaviour is a subtle yet powerful internal conflict, where we unconsciously undermine our healing process, achievements and, by extension, our happiness. Quite frequently this doesn't take place at the conscious level, which means that consciously we all want to get better, to succeed in life and to be happy. At our subconscious level, however, the feeling that we don't "deserve" to be in good health activates a complex mechanism that subverts the normal healing process. What causes this enigmatic behavior?

Mainstream psychology believes that self-sabotage is induced by low self-esteem, which is generally a result of a "bad programme" quite often insidiously planted in early childhood. Remarks like "You are a bad boy" or "You will never succeed in life", carelessly said by an upset parent, can imprint in the child's subconscious mind that he/she is not worthy of happiness. Later on, as an adult, every time the person experiences a sense of wellbeing, an always-alert mechanism is set off carrying the message "I don't deserve to be healthy".

Also, in some cases the person "needs" the health issue in order to be acknowledged and loved, as we have seen before. In both circumstances the outcome is the same: unless the therapist is aware of the situation, the treatment has very little chance of succeeding.

Interestingly, despite being a complex situation with deep roots, which can be responsible for long-lasting ailments, self-sabotage can be efficiently defused just by acknowledging its presence. In other words, once the person becomes aware that he/she is unconsciously sabotaging the healing process, it ceases to exist!

Jerry Kein, a well-known American hypnotherapist, once shared an interesting case involving self-sabotage. Years ago, an attractive lady came to his office looking for help. She had an uncontrollable habit of constantly pulling her hair. Under hypnosis it was found out that as a child she had been repeatedly sexually abused. Therefore, with a low self-worth she started to punish herself by destroying her physical appearance. Once the roots of her problem surfaced and a positive message was suggested under hypnosis, her disfiguring behavior disappeared.

As we have seen before, traumatic or challenging episodes, whether real or imaginary, have the power of leaving scars on our subconscious minds. Chinese wisdom explains this further by saying that traumatic experiences cause energy stagnation in our magnetic field, which is ultimately connected to our vital force.

Chinese medicine considers that feelings of undeserved wellbeing can strongly affect the **Lung's energy**. The Lung-Chi is responsible for the Defensive Chi, which in Western medicine terms can be understood as our immune system. Indeed, people suffering from low self-esteem present shallow breathing and sunken chest, and are prone to auto-immune disorders such as lupus, rheumatoid arthritis, asthma, etc.

Incidentally, the traditional religious habit of hitting one's own chest while saying "*Mea culpa, mea culpa, mea maxima culpa*" can be interpreted as some sort of self-flagellation. The thymus gland, one of the main glands responsible for our immune system is located in the center of our chest, and is also energetically connected to the Lungs. Therefore, hitting the chest with the idea of punishment can send our subconscious mind the message that we don't like ourselves, and can destabilize our energetic system.

Now, whenever I suspect that there is an element of sabotage present, I ask the patient to hold the arm outstraight, at shoulder level, and to say out loud: "I want to get better". I then apply a slight pressure downward on the arm. If the arm remains straight and strong the prospect of recovery is good. However, if I feel any sign of weakness, there is almost certainly an element of self-sabotage present.

PART TWO

Therapies

Colours, Emotions and Chinese Medicine

Acupuncture

Flower Essences

Hands

Stretching

Breathing Techniques

Visualization Techniques

Self-Hypnosis

Chapter VIII

Colours, Emotions and Chinese Medicine

Colours can represent emotions and emotions can manifest themselves through colours. Here are a few examples:

Red = angry, infuriated
Green = envy, jealousy
Blue = melancholy
White = fear
Yellow = cowardly

We are aware, consciously or not, of the effects of colours on our mood. One can feel excited or relaxed, depending on the colours to which one is exposed. Leonardo Da Vinci once said, *"The power of meditation can be ten times greater under a violet light falling through the stained glass window of a quiet church."*

Not long ago, British mental institutions performed an interesting experiment. Individuals displaying signs of aggressiveness were placed in rooms painted with soothing colours, whereas depressive ones were exposed to vibrant ones. The results were very encouraging in both cases: the aggressive ones became more relaxed and the depressive ones became more cheerful.

Another interesting fact proving the power of colours can be found in major fast-food restaurants. They are generally painted with vibrant colours, like orange and red with bright light as well. Let's imagine a fast-food cafeteria tastefully decorated with off-white soothing colours, dim lights and relaxing music. The customer would order his hamburger and French-fries and chew his meal slowly and would tend to stay longer enjoying the peaceful ambiance. However, since the purpose is to sell *fast* food, the idea is to have the person place the order, eat and leave the place as quickly as possible. Here lies the proof of the power of colours implemented by powerful and down-to-earth companies.

Since the dawn of humankind all living beings on the planet have been energized and nurtured by the Sun. The history of civilizations has demonstrated that no matter how primitive people are, there has always been a deep respect and reverence for the Sun. Our ancestors, the cavemen, were naturally aware of the importance and the healing power of sunrays and the myriad of colours resulting from them.

Healing through colours was extensively performed during Greece's Golden Age and at the Healing Temples of Heliopolis, ancient Egypt. It was also revered by ancient civilizations like India and China. In the Egyptian temples, archeologists have found evidence of a special type of construction, where rooms were built so that the sun's rays were broken up into seven colours. The healer would diagnose what colour or colours the individual lacked, and then the patient would be placed in the room bathed by the specific colour he/she needed for the restoration of his/her health. This proves that light and colours were used in the past not only for worship but for healing purposes as well.

In later stages of our civilization there were many artists whose works impress us with vibrant blends of colours, like Da Vinci, Michelangelo, Van Gogh, Gaugin, just to name a few. They were masters in expressing themselves through colours and are responsible for improving our sensitivity and uplifting our spirits.

In modern days we must acknowledge Walt Disney's immense contribution to the world of colours. I compare his work with Mozart's phenomenal music legacy. Mozart with his exceptional talent created melodies and expanded our perception of refined music. Disney did the same thing in the field of colours. They both are responsible for improving our perception of subtler dimensions and softening our hearts.

Modern science contemplates colours as being radiation of a certain length. The sunlight passing through a prism breaks down into seven colours: red, orange, yellow, green, blue, indigo and violet. The colours violet and red representing the extremes of the spectrum are the limits as to how far a human eye can see. It is known, however, that by means of sensitive optical instruments, invisible radiation can be detected showing also infrared and ultraviolet. Moreover, it's known that higher wave-length colours, like red, can be seen from a far distance; that is why red lights are normally used at night in cars' back lights, and on top of towers and buildings.

Eastern philosophy, on the other hand, considers colour as being also a vibration, a healing force. Between two main polarities, light and darkness, colour represents the balance. Neither total light nor total darkness maintains life. According to Goethe (German scientist and poet), *"the birth of colours takes place through the interplay of light and darkness."*

Chinese medicine relies considerably on colours for diagnostic and treatment purposes. The *Nei Jing,* considered to be the most important Chinese medicine text, says: *"Every disease has a symbol amongst the variety of colours."* From the Taoist's Yin/Yang conception, vibrant colours like **red, orange and yellow** are considered to have **Yang** quality, whereas soothing colours like **blue and violet** would be regarded as being **Yin**. Then comes the question, "How about green?" Well, since green results from a blend of yellow (Yang) and blue (Yin), it is considered to be a well-balanced colour, a healing colour *par excellence.*

Considering the relationship of Yin/Yang and colours, the simplest yet most effective form of treatment would be:

a. In cases where strong signs and/or emotions (Yang) are present, like anger, irritation and hyper-activity one should use soothing colours: *blue, violet and purple.*

b. In cases of weak signs and/or low energy emotions (Yin), like guilt, depression, sadness and hypo-activity, colours like *red, yellow and orange* should be applied.

c. In both circumstances the colour *green* should be added to the chosen colour, for it can help stabilize the process.

At the end of this chapter, practical treatment suggestions will be presented.

As we have seen above, together with the Yin/Yang concept, the theory of the Five Elements constitutes the basis of Chinese medicine. Even today with all the technological advances and new developments applied to holistic health care, the Five Elements theory continues to be an important and reliable source of inspiration for modern holistic therapists.

Cases where one or more colours predominate (meaning: the skin showing abnormal colouration, of course taking into account ethnic variety) indicate an imbalance in the corresponding element. For instance:

> Red: Fire imbalance - heat in the Heart
> Yellow: Earth imbalance - Spleen deficiency
> White (pale): Metal imbalance - Lung deficiency
> Dark (grey/black): Water imbalance - Kidney deficiency
> Green: Wood imbalance - Liver problem

Also there can be more complex cases, such as:

- Pale face and red cheeks = Fire (red) element invading Metal (white)
- Yellowish face and a green hue around the mouth = Wood (green) attacking Earth (yellow)

When we are dealing with emotions, the theory of the Five Elements can be a useful tool not only in helping to identify the organ affected, but also in choosing the treatment. When using colours as therapy for emotional disharmony, it is important to take into account that certain emotions are a result of excessive energetic activity of the organs related to them; others are signs of energy deficiency. Again, whenever we are dealing with excesses, we have to *control* or *reduce* them; while in cases of deficiency, we have to *tonify* or *suplement* them.

- When dealing with *anger* (Wood in excess)→ white (Metal) is the colour of choice, for Metal controls Wood;

- When dealing with *impatience* (Fire in excess)→ dark blue or black (Water) are the colours to use, for Water controls Fire;

- When dealing with *worry* (Earth deficiency)→ red (Fire) and yellow (Earth) are the colours of choice, for Fire generates Earth and yellow nurtures Earth;

- When dealing with *fear* (Water deficiency)→ white (Metal) and black or dark blue (Water) are the best colours to use, for Metal generates Water and black/dark blue nurture Water.

- When dealing with *sadness* (Metal deficiency)➔ yellow (Earth) and white (Metal) are the colours of choice, for Earth generates Metal and white nurtures Metal.

The above therapy method is based on the Five Elements' controlling sequence. It is also important to mention that the colours that we always have around us are a strong indication that those are the ones we lack, whereas the ones we reject are the ones we have in excess. This can apply to clothes, cars, flowers, paints, etc. I used to have a patient who couldn't stand the colour yellow and would be outraged at somebody spending a huge amount of money in buying a yellow car. The person had an excess- imbalance in Earth element, where adding more yellow colours would aggravate the problem.

Therapy using colours

There are many ways to use colours as therapy. The most popular ones are the application of coloured light to certain areas of the body with the purpose of increasing or reducing the amount of energy. Normally a variety of coloured light bulbs or coloured filters are applied.

The areas regularly chosen are the *chakras* or the seven energy centers; reflex areas, like hands and feet; or acupuncture points. The latter technique is known as colourpuncture, a system developed by Peter Mandel, which combines colour therapy and meridian theory. Needless to say, it is a technique that requires knowledge of acupuncture and sophisticated equipment.

Interestingly, in 1984, while studying acupuncture in Japan and totally unaware of Mandel's work I conducted some experiments integrating colour therapy and acupuncture. Before diverging my interest to Chinese medicine, I was deeply involved with the use of colours as therapy thanks to the teachings of Rene Nunes, a well-known Brazilian researcher, who dedicated a good deal of his life to humanitarian service through colour therapy. Thus, when acupuncture began to be part of my life, I naturally considered ways of integrating both therapies.

I once adapted a very fine quartz crystal to a small flashlight and through the use of a variety of coloured cellophane paper, I applied different colours to acupuncture points. One day, I remember well, as I was holding the flashlight with a green colour filter over the Liver meridian, I felt a sharp pain under the right ribcage - liver area! That was an amazing sensation, which confirmed the effect of colour in the flow of Chi. I strongly believe that in the future acupuncture will evolve into more subtle forms, using light and sound (vibrations), as our bodies will become less dense. Actually, this is already happening!

In my opinion, it is not by chance that there is a variety of energy oriented therapies today. The main reason for this new paradigm in medicine is because our bodies have become more susceptible and open to subtle therapies. Acupuncture, for instance, has been considered a reliable therapeutic tool by mainstream medicine institutions; the use of magnets has become so widespread for chronic pain treatment, that even the most conventional department stores carry them in all sizes and shapes. Besides, hospitals in the United States are now hiring Reiki practitioners for stress management of post-surgery patients, a situation that would be considered unthinkable a few decades ago.

Anyway, back to colour therapy. Besides the use of sophisticated equipment adopted by many therapists, my experience suggests that there are simpler and no less effective ways to apply colour as therapy.

1. colour-solarized water :

The easiest way of applying colour therapy is by using nature's own abundant light resource: the Sun. The procedure is very simple.

Fill a coloured and transparent container - like a bottle or a jug - with filtered water and exposed it to direct sunlight. If a coloured container is not available, a transparent bottle wrapped with dyed cellophane paper may be used. The light passing through the filter charges the water with the radiation of that particular colour. On a sunny day, one hour of exposure is enough to charge the water, whereas cloudy days would require about three hours. Once charged with the desired colour, the water can be used for any purpose: drinks, teas, etc. When used as therapy it is recommended that the water should be drunk every other week, until the desired results are achieved.

I recommend a very interesting experiment. Place different coloured glasses under sunlight for a while. Then, with the eyes closed, drink a little bit of the water from each one of them and you might be surprised to notice that different colours will have a "different taste". By drinking water that has been charged with a particular colour, one can experience a concentrated form of energy that acts in harmonizing the body, the mind and the emotions.

I normally prescribe this method for my patients as homework or whenever somebody calls from a distant place asking for help. I have had many interesting cases where this therapy alone was enough to solve the problem, such as *yellow* coloured water for babies with *digestive disorders* (like pain, gas); also *yellow* coloured water for *diabetic* patients to help with digestive discomfort; *green* water for *liver*-related problems (like hangover, headaches); *blue* water for children with *sleeping problems*; *orange* water for *depressed* patients, just to name a few.

The most important aspects of the colour-Solarized Water are that it is simple, easy to do, it doesn't require any special skills and we are tapping into nature's inexhaustible resources. The only obstacle is the belief that because it is an uncomplicated method it is worthless. Actually, this is a very common assumption in Western minds accustomed to highly technological devices and gadgets. Unfortunately, despite all scientific advances humankind is still suffering from imbalances not only in the physical body but also from emotional pains. Maybe we lost our sensitivety and wisdom to heal ourselves when the first stethoscope was invented - we began to rely only on equipment, not in our senses. Thus don't let this easy and natural method mislead you. Try it, be adventurous!

2. colours and food

Another form of using the energy of colours is by adopting a therapeutic diet, in which the foods are chosen based on their colour. As with all coloured elements in nature, fruits and vegetables absorb the light radiated by the sun and reflect a certain colour. The food is then saturated with the energy it reflects. Thus, by ingesting colour-charged food we are taking in a very powerful energetic source.

There is, however, a misunderstanding as to what colour a certain food is charged with. Take a watermelon, for instance; is it the outside green peel or the red interior pulp? The answer is, whenever you think of a watermelon, which colour comes first to your mind? Which one impresses you the most? The red, isn't it? How about a banana? Normally the colour which impresses us the most is the yellow peel, not the white pulp. That is a good way to *perceive* the radiation of a certain food.

Here are examples of foods with their respective colours and their therapeutic application in emotional problems.

- Red (or Orange):	tomato, persimmon, strawberry, red pepper, orange, tangerine, watermelon, beets, radish and other fruits, vegetables and seeds in which red or orange predominates. **Therapy**: worry, preoccupation
- Yellow:	pineapple, butter, corn, carrot, pumpkin, mango, melon, peach, papaya, egg yolk, yellow pepper and other fruits, vegetables and seeds in which yellow predominates. **Therapy**: sadness, melancholy and depression
- White:	onions, garlic, horseradish, mushroom, rice, milk and other fruits, vegetables and seeds in which white predominates. **Therapy**: fear, insecurity.
- Black:	black beans, black sesame seeds, seaweed, dark skinned grapes and other fruits, vegetables and seeds in which black, dark purple or dark blue predominate. In terms of Chinese medicine black and blue have similar effects. **Therapy**: impatience, restlessness
- Green:	green coloured vegetables, fruits and seeds. **Therapy**: helps stabilize all the emotions; pacifies the mind

It is also important to add that the colours red, orange and yellow produce an alkaline effect in the body, while blue, navy blue and violet produce an acidic effect.

Besides emotional disorders, there are some physical problems that can be treated by or benefit from certain colours, such as:

- Red:	palpitations, shallow breathing, poor memory, pallor, spontaneous perspiration.
- Yellow:	diarrhea, emaciation, anorexia, edema, hemorrhage, anal prolapse, hernia, muscular atrophy, loss of taste.
- White:	weak voice, respiratory problems, cough, nasal congestion, colds, bronchitis, facial edema.

- **Black**
(or navy blue): frequent urination, impotence, feminine sterility, early ejaculation, vertigo, heat sensation in the palms of the hands and the soles of the feet, tinnitus.

- **Green**:
irregular menstruation, eye problems, joint problems, brittle nails.

- **Violet**:
nervous and mental disorders, neurosis, neuralgia, sciatica, scalp diseases, epilepsy, cramps, rheumatism, cataracts.

- **Blue**
(powerful antiseptic): throat problems, laryngitis, goiter, hoarseness, fever, mouth ulcers, acute rheumatism, strokes.

The Yogic tradition (India) has also an interesting approach to colours, food and the Zodiac signs. Although I am not an expert in astrology, I thought this would be extra information for those who are.

Aquarius:
Aquarians lack the colours blue and white; their bodies work better on a diet of blue and white fruits and vegetables, like grapes, pears, asparagus, celery, mung beans, alfafa sprouts, potato (in moderation), horse- radish, fish and chicken. The Aquarians have problems digesting starch, like pasta, macaroni, spaghetti.

Pisces:
the natives of this sign lack the colours green and white; the recommended foods are roots (vegetables), fruits and vegetables, fish, chicken and eggs. The Pisceans are prone to problems with lymph glands, feet and emotions.

Aries:
the natives of Aries lack red: red pepper, strawberry, tomato, radish, watermelon, red meat. They are prone to head injuries, headaches, hypertension.

Taurus:
the natives of this sign lack yellow: carrots, melon, corn, butter. They need large amounts of vitamin A

and C. They are prone to weight, thyroid and throat problems.

Gemini: the Geminians lack the colours purple and yellow; they need foods rich in both of those colours. They are prone to nervous system problems, fractures (hands, arms, shoulders) and are shallow breathers.

Cancer: people born in cancer lack the colours white and green; their bodies react well to foods rich in both colours, specially those cultivated in the shade or in indirect sunlight, like cucumber, melon, squash. The Cancerians are prone to digestion system problems, cataracts and glaucoma.

Leo: the natives of this sign lack the colours yellow and orange. They need large quantities of vitamin C. The recommended foods are: melon, pumpkin, squash. The natives of Leo are prone to circulatory and heart problems.

Virgo: the Virginians lack the colours violet and gold. They need grains and foods rich in Potassium. They have a tendency towards pancreas problems (diabetes), liver disorders and diarrhea due to stress.

Libra: Librians lack the colours gold and crimson. They need red and yellow fruits and vegetables, specially the ones grown above the ground. The natives of Libra are prone to eliminatory system disharmony, like kidneys, liver and skin problems.

Scorpio: those born in this sign lack the colours red and scarlet. They need to drink large amounts of liquid; so they need juicy yellow and red fruits and vegetables. Fiber intake and exercise are highly recommended. These individuals have lots of energy but are prone to large intestine problems (constipation) and problems with the reproductive system.

***Sagittarius*:**   the natives of this sign lack the colours red and gold and are normally deficient in enzymes. They need red and golden foods, especially raw. The Sagittarians are prone to sciatic nerve and hip region problems and are also shallow breathers.

***Capricorn*:**   the natives of this sign lack the colours green and black. Foods that have enough of these colours, like roots and seaweed are recommended. They are prone to liver, gallbladder and knee problems and have difficulty in expressing emotions.

Chapter IX

Acupuncture

Whenever acupuncture is the subject of a conversation, it is quite common to hear: "Doesn't it hurt?" or "I don't want to be looking like a porcupine with all those needles inserted in me!" or "Needles? Not me. I'd much rather take my drugs!" These are, of course, comments made by someone who has never had the opportunity to experience acupuncture.

Acupuncture is perhaps the most popular therapy of Chinese medicine. Its wide range of action and effectiveness has been challenging Western science for centuries, and that is precisely the point: only a potent and effective therapeutic method would have survived all these centuries, basically intact. In Japan, acupuncture is considered not only a therapy but also an art. Its practice requires skill, precision and refinement. The needles are very fine (some of them are as thick as a hair) and some acupuncturists have reached such a degree of mastery and barely insert them.

The earliest records on acupuncture date back to 2.600 BC, in China, but archeological findings suggest that its practice goes further back in time. There is evidence that the practice of piercing the skin for therapeutic purposes was not limited to Asia, but was also present in ancient Egypt, Persia and amongst the indigenous of Brazil. Egyptologists are aware that in ancient times, the Egyptians used to pierce the ears for healing purposes (they were perhaps the first ones to wear earrings). Interestingly, on my trip to Egypt in 1988, I was quite surprised to see a painting depicting a scene of somebody being treated with acupuncture at the temple of Kom Ombo, on the Nile.

Why do you think the pirates are normally portrayed wearing one earring? Was it only for adornment purposes? There is always a good reason for everything and this case is no exception. The main reason is that in the old days there weren't optical instruments, like binoculars or lunettes available and, since the pirates needed to have sharp vision to spot their victims, they used to pierce the center of one earlobe: the eye point! The Persians, who in the old days were famous for their medicine, used to insert pieces of metal in the body for therapeutic purposes. Moreover, there are accounts of Brazilian Indians piercing their bodies with thorns and fishbones to drive out evil spirits, "the ultimate cause of diseases". These facts prove that knowledge is universal and has common roots. By looking back at the history of humankind we see different ethnic groups, totally isolated from one another with similar habits, ideas and rituals.

However, despite historical records showing the practice of acupuncture by other ethnical groups, the Chinese were the ones who created what we know as acupuncture today. They have developed a whole therapy system based on the insertion of fine needles in certain points of the body. Some scholars believe that in the beginning, piercing the skin with very fine stones or needles made of bamboo was part of shamanic practices; disease was believed to be an act of angry gods. It is known, however, that the careful detailed observation and interpretation of nature's phenomena were the basic foundation of Chinese philosophy and medicine.

The ancient Chinese observed the presence of tender points in specific parts of the skin whenever an individual came down with a health problem, regardless of the area of its manifestation. For instance, they observed that someone complaining of headache would also present tender spots in the feet! Moreover, warriors who were wounded by arrows in battles experienced relief of symptoms of their illness. By associating those tender points and wounded areas to certain diseases, the early Chinese realized that they formed a distinct pattern of lines all over the body. These lines were later called "meridians" or "channels", through which Chi or life force flows, as we have seen in previous pages.

How can acupuncture treat emotional disorders? As we have seen before, the energetic aspect of the main organs manifests externally through a particular emotion. A person who is angry all the time could be suffering from Liver hyper-function, which can be an early sign of a "real" Liver disorder. "Real" here means a disease detectable by conventional medicine. Therefore, in this case the person is bound to present some disturbance in the energy flow, like tender points along the meridians detectable by palpation, pulse and tongue examination, etc. Thus, once the blockages and the meridian or meridians involved are located, the acupuncturists decide the best approach to the case. That can be the use of acupuncture alone or, most commonly, a combination of needles, herbs, massage and dietary suggestions.

I have treated cases of depression by using a combination of acupuncture, Chinese herbs and hypnotherapy, which will be discussed later on. It is important to be flexible and to be open to the individual's needs. However, since the majority of people diagnosed as suffering from depression also present stagnation of Liver-Chi, the best approach is to use all the methods that help to free Chi. It is also very important to **listen.** Quite often by sharing our inner problems with somebody we trust, we experience a considerable relief; therefore, a therapist should put aside some time to just listen to what goes on in his patient's heart.

My experience also recommends that whenever we are dealing with an emotional disorder such as depression, it is better to concentrate on the energy aspect of the case; meaning, removing the blockages and coursing the Chi, according to the pattern or patterns present in the case. Sometimes, especially in the beginning of the treatment, the individual is so caught up in his/her own suffering and the mind is so blurred that trying to access the person's intellectual area by questioning and reasoning may prove to be fruitless. Once the mind is pacified through acupuncture treatment, that would be the time to ask those questions, not before.

Ear acupuncture is a very effective method of acupuncture, for it can play an important role when it comes to treating nervous-related disorders, and controlling appetite and drug (also alcohol and smoking) addiction. This kind of acupuncture works on reflex areas as opposed to systemic (whole body) acupuncture, which contemplates meridians. Nevertheless, in the case of a physical or emotional disorder, one can detect and treat sensitive points on the surface of the ear. There are points, for instance, that can induce the brain to release endorphins, substances responsible for sensations of well being, pain alleviation and relaxation. Although maps of ear acupuncture were first published in China in 1950, the French carried on with deep and important studies in the field.

It is also very important to understand that when dealing with an emotional disturbance, there is no such thing as an immediate result. It is not like taking a pill which has quick results but only controls the problem; it does not cure it. Holistic therapies, like acupuncture, work with the person; the problem is just a reference. Therefore, there are some steps to be taken, and they are basically a "process" in which all the aspects of the individual (mind, body and emotion) are taken into consideration. The only way to get to the core of an onion is by taking off layer after layer.

From the Chinese medicine perspective, there are some symptoms or signs that are important energetic indicators of which organ or organs are being affected. "If one wants to know what goes on inside, look for exterior manifestations."

- Feeling down, rootless and weak → treat Spleen
- Sadness, melancholy and quiet → Lungs
- Fearful and insecure → Kidneys
- Weak voice → Lungs and Large Intestine
- Can't make up his/her mind; indecision; can't carry on with plans → Gall Bladder;
- Occasional emotional outbursts → Liver
- Lack of courage; timidity → Gall Bladder
- Impatience; restlessness → Heart
- Sees the world as being "grey" → Liver
- Oppression in the chest; sensation of "something stuck in the throat" → Liver
- Life feels as if "I am driving with the hand-brake on" → Liver
- Mental confusion; disorientation; absent mindedness → Heart
- Excess jealousy; suspicion → Gall Bladder
- Talks non stop → Heart
- Lethargy; sunken eyes → Spleen
- Tiredness; bags or dark colour under eyes → Kidneys
- Irritation; mood swings → Stomach
- Lack of flexibility; perfectionism → Spleen
- Ruminating; worrying → Spleen
- Feelings of frustration; unfulfilled desires → Liver
- Excessive joy (hysteria) → Heart
- Shock; trauma → Kidneys and Heart
- Incapacity of sound judgement; lack of mental clarity → Small Intestine
- Problems with space (agoraphobia or claustrophobia) → Lungs
- Feeling of oppression from people around → Lungs
- Uncomfortable in parties, meetings, speaking in public → Lungs

Chapter X

Flower Essences

Flower Essences are perhaps, one of the most effective therapeutic tools when dealing with emotional issues. They are herbal infusions or decoctions made from flowers, where the flower's vibrational force is transferred to water in a process similar to homeopathy. The flowers are picked, placed floating in a glass bowl filled with water and left exposed to the sun for a while. The water will then be printed with the flower's energy qualities.

Vibrational medicine like flower essences is part of many ancient cultures throughout the world. The XVI century Swiss physician and alchemist Paracelsus (Theophrastus Bombastus von Hohenheim), whose work marks the beginning of the emergence of chemistry from alchemy, is considered one of the pioneers of homeopathy and flower essence therapy.

The best known precursor of flower essence therapy in the modern world is the English physician, Dr. Edward Bach, a renowned bacteriologist, pathologist and homeopath. His orthodox research resulted in a series of oral vaccines known as Bach Nosodes. A Nosode is a homeopathic remedy prepared from a pathological specimen, such as blood, pus, any body secretion or excretion, a diseased fragment of tissue, etc. A nosode could be described as an "oral vaccine", since its purpose is to immunize the body against a specific disease.

Even though his work received great acclaim, Bach was not satisfied. He considered that the vaccines could be replaced by plants, which he believed to be more effective. Guided by his enthusiasm and scientific spirit he left behind his prestigious carrier, closed his clinic and moved to the countryside. The story goes that he packed all his medical instruments in a suitcase, only to find out later on upon arriving to his destination, that he had brought a case full of shoes instead! Thus, the only "instruments" he had to work with were careful and patient observation and intuition.

Bach had always been more interested in the people suffering from a disease than in the disease itself, a fact that brings his concept very close to Chinese medicine's foundations. As previously discussed, one of the most important aspects of Chinese medicine is that body, mind and emotion should be taken equally into account. The attention should be given to the individual, not to his disease. Thus, by working with flower essences, Bach was equally convinced that true health could only be maintained by treating the individual personality, instead of concentrating on the body's diseases.

Upon working with flower essences, Bach found out that when properly administrated according to the personality and emotional states of individuals, he could solve these imbalances and clear the ground for the physical ailments to heal as well. At the time of his death in 1936, Bach had discovered 38 remedies suitable to treat every possible emotional issue, with each individual remedy or a combination of some of them.

The 38 original Bach Flower Essences are:

1. **Agrimony:** for those who hide worries behind a brave face

2. **Aspen:** for people who are anxious or afraid but don't know why

3. **Beech:** for those who are critical and intolerant of others

4. **Centaury:** for people who allow others to impose on them

5. **Cerato:** those who doubt their own judgement

6. **Cherry Plum:** uncontrolled, irrational thoughts and the fear of doing something awful.

7. **Chestnut Bud :** for those who repeat the same mistakes and don't learn from them.

8. **Chicory:** for over-possessive, selfish people who cling to their loved ones

9. **Clematis:** for day-dreamers, absent-minded people

10. **Crab Apple**: for those who dislike the way they look, and as a general cleanser

11. **Elm:** for capable people who in a crisis doubt their ability to cope

12. **Gentian:** for those easily disheartened when something goes wrong

13. **Gorse:** for pessimism, defeatism

14. **Heather:** for people who are talkative and obsessed with their own problems

15. **Holly:** for feelings of hatred, envy, jealously and suspicion

16. **Honeysuckle:** for those who live in the past

17. **Hornbeam:** for people who find it difficult to face everyday problems, procrastination .

18. **Impatiens:** for impatience and irritation at other people's slowness

19. **Larch:** for fear of failure and lack of confidence

20. **Mimulus:** for those who fear something real that they can name

21. **Mustard:** for gloom and depression with no known cause

22. **Oak:** for strong people who can over-extend themselves by trying too hard

23. **Olive:** for those physically drained by exertion or illness

24. **Pine:** for people who blame themselves when things go wrong; guilt

25. **Red Chestnut:** for excessive worry about the welfare of loved ones

26. **Rock Rose:** for extreme fright and terror

27. Rock Water: for people who are excessively self-disciplined; rigid minded

28. Scleranthus: for those who find it difficult to choose between possible courses of action.

29. Star of Bethlehem: for all the effects of serious news, or fright following an accident.

30. Sweet Chestnut: for complete dispair and anguish

31. Vervain: for over-enthusiasm; fanatical beliefs

32. Vine: for domineering people

33. Walnut: assists in adjustment to transition or change, e.g. puberty, menopause, divorce.

34. Water Violet: for reserved and private people, who can appear to be proud and arrogant.

35. White Chestnut: for persistent and worrying thoughts

36. Wild Oat: for those unable to find direction for their lives

37. Wild Rose: for those who resign themselves without complaint; apathy

38. Willow: for those who are full of self-pity, resentment and bitterness

39. Rescue Remedy: for emergency and stressful situations - it is a combination of five essences: Cherry Plum, Clematis, Impatiens, Rock Rose, Star of Bethlehem.

In my practice I always try to understand mental issues from the Chinese medicine perspective. That is a very useful approach, because once you determine which area or areas of the body is/are being affected by the imbalance, it is possible to choose the correct therapy. The most important aspect to be understood is the following relationship or equation:

Negative emotion → Organ disharmony → Negative emotion

Thus, whenever one faces such a vicious cycle it is important to break it in order to bring about healing. The best approach is to work with the subtle and underlying cause: an energy imbalance or, in other words, harmonizing the flow of Chi. Flower essences are a major tool when one aims to course the energy flow regardless of the nature of the imbalance. The following lines show some of the Bach Flower Essences superimposed by the Chinese medicine approach.

Agrimony: (hiding worries) → Earth and Water elements; the stress caused by the effort in disguising the emotion-*worry* (Spleen) depletes Kidney-Chi.

Aspen: (fear and anxiety) → Water and Fire elements; *fear* damages Kidney-Chi and anxiety is the result of lack of "communication" between Water and Fire (Heart).

Beech: (criticism and intolerance) → Fire; those are typical emotions of an imbalance in Heart-Chi.

Centaury:(allowing other's impositions) → Metal element; the Lung's energy manifestation concerns how we relate to exterior conditions like places and people. Not being able to keep one's own space and allowing others to invade it, indicates Lung-Chi deficiency.

Cerato: (doubting one's own judgement) → Fire element; incapacity of sound judgement and lack of mental clarity show Small Intestine-Chi disharmony.

Cherry Plum:(uncontrolled, irrational thoughts) → Wood and Fire elements; outbursts and lack of control point to Liver-Chi hyperfunction, whereas irrational thoughts show signs of Heart-Chi disharmony. As we know, Heart is the "seat of the mind".

Chicory: (over-possessive)

→ Earth element; clinging to loved ones shows Spleen deficiency. The person lacks emotional "nurturing"; needy.

Clematis: (day-dreamers)

→ Fire element; absent-mindedness is a sign of Heart-Chi imbalance.

Crab Apple (poor self-image)

→Metal element; not being happy with the way one manifests exteriorly is a sign of Lung-Chi deficiency. Lung rules the skin.

Gentian (easily disheartened)

→Fire and Water elements imbalance; Heart and Kidney not communicating properly; Heart fails to send Fire to the Kidney.

Gorse (pessimism, defeatism)

→ Water element; Kidney-Chi deficiency manifests itself through lack of will power.

Heather (talkativeness and obsession)

→ Fire element; Heart controls speech and talking non-stop is a sign of excess. Obsession and any other mind-related disturbance are also a sign of Heart-Yang excess (Fire).

Holly (hatred, jealousy, suspicion)

→ Wood and Fire elements; jealousy and suspicion are related to Gall Bladder imbalance, whereas hatred as opposite to Love is a sign of Heart disharmony.

Hornbeam (procrastination)

→ Earth element; finding it difficult to face everyday problems is a sign of Spleen deficiency; lack of energy.

Impatiens (impatience)

→ Fire element; impatience and restlessness are typical signs of Heart desharmony.

Larch (fear of failure)

→ Water element; fear of failure and lack of confidence indicate Kidney deficiency; lack of stamina.

Mimulus (fear of something real)

→Water and Fire elements; fear is a sign of Kidney deficiency, which can cause Heart-Chi excess.

Mustard (depression)

→ Wood element; depression indicates energy stagnation, which can be directly or indirectly related to Liver. In Chinese medicine Liver is responsible for ensuring the smooth flow of Chi.

Olive (exhaustion)

→ Earth and Water elements; exhaustion, physical drain indicate Spleen and Kidney deficiency.

Pine (guilt)

→ Fire and Water elements; guilt affects the Heart and the Kidney and causes Chi to stagnate in the chest, epigastrium or abdomen.

Red Chestnut (worry)

→ Earth element; excessive worry damages Spleen.

Rock Rose (extreme fright)

→ Fire and Water elements; extreme fear injures the Kidneys and causes the Mind (Heart) to be out of control.

Rock Water (rigidity)

→ Earth element; lack of flexibility is related to Spleen imbalance.

Scleranthus (indecision)

→ Wood element; indecision is a common sign of Gall Bladder disharmony.

Star of Bethlehem (shock)

→ Water and Fire elements; shock scatters Chi and affects the Heart and the Kidneys.

Sweet Chestnut (dispair)

→ Fire and Water elements; dispair and anguish drain Kidney's energy and consequently disturbs the Mind (Heart).

Vervain (over-enthusiasm)

→ Fire element; enthusiasm is normally a positive state of mind but excess of excitement can injure the Heart.

Water Violet (quiet and privacy)

→ Metal element; difficulty in interacting with other people and preference for isolation indicate Lung deficiency.

White Chestnut (persistent worry)

→ Earth and Metal elements; worry depletes Spleen and also "knots" Lung-Chi.

Wild Oat (unable to find direction) → Wood element; inability to find direction for one's life is a sign of Gall Bladder deficiency.

Wild Rose (apathy) →Metal and Earth elements; apathy, lack of strength to fight indicate Spleen and Lung deficiency.

Willow (resentment and bitterness) →Fire and Wood elements; resentment causes Liver-Chi stagnation; whereas bitterness indicates Heart disharmony.

The above mentioned essences are not the only ones available. They are just the ones I am more familiar with. Dr.Bach's legacy was carried on by many researchers who developed an amazing number and variety of flower essences. I will mention some: FES - Flower Essence Society, from California, Alaskan Flower Essences, Desert Flower Essences, Australian F. Essences, Hawaiian, Florais de Minas (Brazil), Findhorn Foundation (Scotland), Canadian and many others.

The most fascinating aspect of the newly developed flower essences is that many of them are geared not only to emotional or mental disharmony, but also to physical problems as well.

Chapter XI

Hands

Besides our facial muscles, no other part of the human anatomy expresses emotions as perfectly as the hands. Our hands, with a wide range of gestures and movements, are capable of conveying our thoughts and our feelings in a precise and detailed way. Crisp hands and tight fists signify tension and anger; shaking hands mean fear; perspiring hands and "nervous" hands reveal worry and so forth.

The Chinese believe that the hands are an extension of the Heart, and since the Heart is considered to be the seat of the Mind, it is understandable that gentle and harmonious gestures reflect a peaceful heart. On the other hand, a disturbed Heart (Mind) is the underlying cause behind aggressive, agitated and uncontrolled hand movements.

Throughout our lives we rely on our hands to perform a myriad of functions that range from basic skills, like feeding ourselves to the most subtle and elevated expressions of our being, like healing and praying. The highly sensitive nerve endings that irrigate the whole surface of the hands are responsible for one of the human being's most basic and refined senses - the tactile sense.

The human tactile sense is so refined that it can compensate for the absence of sight, as in the case of the blind, who develop an amazing capacity of "seeing" through their hands. In Japan there is a well-known acupuncture school for the blind and they are famous for their skill and technique - their tactile sense is so accurate that they can diagnose and administer the treatment with precision. The school carries on with a long tradition that goes back to the seventeenth century

84

AD. During the shogunate period, the warriors or samurais were considered to be a very high and honorable profession. The story goes that a samurai's son who was getting prepared to follow his father's footsteps, suffered an accident and became blind. Understandably, the episode was devastating to the youngster for, all of a sudden, the dream of becoming a samurai crumbled to pieces. However, as time went by, he developed a remarkable massage skill, that led the Shogun not only to appoint him as his personal therapist but also to open the first therapy school for the blind.

While in Japan, I was exposed to a great variety of therapy techniques that require considerable hand skills, like abdominal and pulse diagnosis; a single-handed needle insertion in acupuncture treatment; special massage strokes in shiatsu, just to name a few. Hand skills are a praised activity nationwide. The masters of any traditional handicraft techniques like basket making, lacquerware painting, woodcarving, papermaking and others are considered to be "National Living Treasures".

Interestingly, in Japan, *ikebana* (flower arrangement), *origami* (paper folding) and calligraphy are included in the training activities of policemen. These handicraft techniques are considered to be important in the development of sensitivity and also help to soften the character. Thus, the same hands that are trained to break bricks can carefully blend flowers in a delicate arrangement!

From the energetic perspective, the hands are the terminal points for all the meridians that flow to or from the fingers. By working with the hands, we are certainly stimulating the energy channel network that circulates all over our body. There are certain points in the hands, however, that are closely associated with the Liver and the Heart , which are according to Chinese medicine, responsible for the "absorption" and the manifestation of the emotions, respectively. That could explain why people suffering from tension and stress experience a deep sensation of well being when working with the hands such as gardening, pottery, carpentry and handicrafts in general. In summary, by working with the hands we are expressing our feelings exteriorly and simultaneously harmonizing our emotions internally as well. In the following lines we shall explore the therapeutic effect of handicrafts.

Origami

Although Origami is a Japanese word for the art of paper folding (*ori,* to fold and *kami,* paper), its origin is unknown. The technique of papermaking was introduced to Japan from China during the early seventh century by Buddhist missionaries. In the beginning, paper was exclusively reserved for religious purposes such as ceremonies and the transcript of sutras. Later on, with the improvement and increased availability of paper, it was used for more mundane purposes like bags, kites, lanterns, umbrellas and screens. Even nowadays, there are traditional papermakers in Japan who perform the same refined technique passed on through generations by their ancestors.

In 1985, I went to visit one of those "living treasures" of papermaking in the Kansai province. I remember it very well; it was a simple wooden house with partitions made of rice paper. At the entrance, I was welcomed by a smiling old man who proceeded to show me his workshop. There, I saw a middle-aged lady bending over a tank filled up with a whitish liquid, while holding a large frame. It was a very interesting scene because she looked as though she was performing a rhythmic dance. In one motion, she would immerse the frame in a forward movement and then to the right and the left like a pendulum. The idea was to allow the fibers to be interwoven on the frame. After a while, she would turn the frame upside down over a wide wooden board and a white thick layer of wet paper would be left to dry. Later on, I asked the master how long it would take to be proficient in the papermaking technique. He thought for a moment and said with a smile, "Fifty years!"

Even though it is not clear when paper folding became a form of art in Japan, by the seventeenth century, with the well-regulated lifestyle brought about by the advent of samurai society, Origami flourished. It was first used for formal purposes but later on paper folding started to be practiced for pure enjoyment and therapeutic purposes, i.e. a channel for emotions during illnesses or misfortunes. During the Meiji period (1868-1912), when Japan started to establish trade connections with foreign countries, Japanese art and culture were also well received abroad including Origami. However, the use of Origami as therapy is the main object of our attention in this present work.

The art of paper folding has been used for therapeutic purposes in Western countries since the beginning of the twentieth century. It has proven to be very effective for the following:

- dealing with mental health patients, the handicapped, prisoners; treating drug addicts; in occupational therapy, in rehabilitation of hands after surgery, in children with ADHD; treating anxiety, stress and aggression, and in cases of autism.

The outstanding advantage of Origami is that it can be used as a form of non-verbal communication, conveying the feeling of acceptance in a group, and promoting the sense of achievement -"it is one's own creation, something one has total control over". It also has the capacity of breaking the ice and can be used as bridging therapy. As John Morin states in his book *The Ultimate Origami Book*, "through Origami, you discover more about yourself. The origamist leaves a piece of himself in every model he creates…As you shape a sheet of paper into a finished model, the paper, in turn, shapes you. The paper in front of you takes on a life of its own."

J.C. Trewin, in his book *Tutor to the Tsarevitch,* mentions an interesting case where paper folding was used with success by a tutor in an attempt to communicate with a nine-year-old boy who was incapable of interacting with the exterior world. Through careful and patient effort, the tutor taught the boy how to make hats using paper-folding art. He got so stimulated by his achievement that he started not only to communicate but also to interact with other children, as well. There are also many records of doctors, nurses, art therapists and teachers applying "Origami Therapy" in their field of action with remarkable positive results.*

What I find fascinating in Origami is that, by working on certain models or forms, we can not only experience a great sense of achievement, but also relaxation and emotional healing. In Japan, it is tradition to fold cranes for someone who is sick, since cranes are revered symbols of longevity and good health. Other models of forms convey very special meanings, such as:

-   swan → love, peace and beauty
-   fish (carp) → reverence, sacredness
-   windmill → joy
-   butterfly → lightness
-   flower → purity
-   sailboat → freedom
-   box → symbolically used to carry one's problems (it is thrown in a stream to be taken away).
-   crane → longevity and good health
-   phoenix → inspiration, vision, conveys the sense of "rising from the aches" after misfortunes
-   turtle → security, stability
-   tiger → defense, protection, strength
-   dragon → wisdom, power

Thus, when dealing with emotional issues, one can effectively draw from the power of the forms and shapes of Origami models. By creating a form that is paradoxically opposite to the problem, we are offering others and ourselves a potent antidote.

* There are nowadays many Origami clubs and associations formed by Origami enthusiasts, which can be contacted on the Internet.

Calligraphy

Archeological findings have proven that since the dawn of humankind, we have been trying our best to express our thoughts and feelings through a wide variety of symbols, carefully and systematically drawn on caves, stones, clay tablets, temple walls and columns, animal skins, papyrus and more recently, on paper.

The ancient Egyptians were particularly prolific in writing details about their lives for posterity. Thanks to all the symbols and drawings painted or carved mainly on walls, we now have a wealth of information about their lives, customs and beliefs. The hieroglyphs are capable of bringing to life echoes of a civilization lost thousands of years ago. Each symbol carries the energy imprinted in it by the writer.

The ancient Chinese also developed a system of writing, which was primarily based on symbolic language. The characters originated between 2000 - 1500 B.C in the Yellow River region of China. In the beginning they were mostly simple pictographs, but with time became increasingly more complex and abstract, consequently foreign students of the Chinese language are soon faced with a major challenge: the characters represent not only sound, but also images. Therefore, whenever a translation is made it is important that one takes into account that a text carries much more than characters tied up together; it includes the author's feelings and energy imprinted in it.

Migrating Chinese and Koreans brought the Chinese characters to Japan around the fourth century AD. In that period, the Japanese language existed only in spoken form and the *kanji* (the Japanese word that means "symbols of China") were borrowed to enable it to be expressed in written form. Today the written Japanese language contains three basic characters: the kanji or Chinese ideographs, *hiragana* - Japanese phonetic figures, and *katakana,* created to express Western languages.

Sho or Japanese calligraphy is a highly appreciated art form, where a single character or words are drawn following established principles of stroke order. They are created with a special brush, ink and paper and their beauty lies in the power generated by each brush stroke as it takes form on the paper. The Japanese believe that by practicing calligraphy one develops the two sides of the brain simultaneously, for it involves both emotion and precision.

More that an art form, Japanese Calligraphy can be a powerful therapeutic tool especially where emotions are concerned. It is a direct reflection of the artist's contemporary concerns as well as being an expression of the individual's identity and feelings.

In the ancient city of Nara, there is a group of artists with physical and learning disabilities called "Group Monji-Ya" (literally *wordsmiths*). For the past eight years under the guidance of the calligrapher Meyio Miami, they have been encouraged to express their feelings by using the brush, ink and paper as their medium. Their work is so intense that it has captured the hearts of the Japanese. The calligraphers channel their emotions by creating one character that they may never be able to draw again, and that creates the maximum intensity of passion with a minimum amount of expression.

The Japanese have an old custom of asking children to write the phrase "Be careful with fire" using brush and ink and displaying it in the kitchen. It is believed that children's writing has the power to prevent fire. This belief demonstrates what the Japanese call the "Spirit of Figures", the "magical" power of calligraphy as the writing of innocent children energizes it.

Pottery

Have you ever wondered why people say that they experience a great feeling of relaxation whenever their work with the hands? Working in the garden, knitting, carpentry and other similar activities have the ability to relax a busy and stressed mind. The explanation could be found in the Chinese medicine concept of energy channels. As explained before, the Chinese maintain that there is an energy network system throughout our body called "meridians". With few exceptions, each of these meridians is connected to an organ and they flow to or from the hands or feet.

Whenever we work with our hands, we necessarily activate some of the energy channels, specially the Pericardium that flows from the chest to the hands. This meridian is not only associated with the heart, as it is understood by mainstream medicine, but it is also connected to the Liver meridian. Both Pericardium and Liver are strongly related to mind and emotions on different levels. Thus, that is one of the reasons why by working with our hands we experience a real sensation of peace and well-being.

One of the most effective handicraft activities for therapy purposes is pottery. Handling the clay, kneading it and creating a form triggers a powerful therapeutic response in us. There is even a therapy for mental and emotional imbalances called "Pottery Therapy". The promoters of this form of therapy believe that the way we handle the clay, our attitude towards the whole process and even the shape that the vessel takes reveal profound nuances of our personality.

Perhaps more than all other crafts, pottery has significantly captured the Japanese spirit: perfectionism, aesthetics and refinement. The clay, the forming process, the tools, the decoration techniques, the glazes, the kiln and fire all have their own modes of expression. The Japanese potter endeavours to allow these individual elements and expressions to emerge. As in the tea ceremony or a traditional Japanese meal, not only the tea and the food are savoured, but the vessels are admired as well. A vessel serves as a "picture frame" for food and is also appreciated on its own. Thus, the wares in which a Japanese meal is served provide nourishment to every aspect of the human psyche: the body, emotions and the mind.

It is important to notice that we instantly associate handling clay, folding paper or drawing with childhood's happy and careless moments. Maybe by manipulating our hands in a creative and oriented way, we can tap into a basic and uncomplicated area of our brain, which, without judgement, allows all our emotions and feelings to emerge in the most varied forms, shapes and colours. Therefore, it doesn't really matter if you have mastered a particular art form, like Japanese calligraphy, Origami or a particular refined pottery style. From the therapist's point of view, it is important to let the hands convey the whole spectrum of our emotions through art, whatever that is. It is literally a "hands-on process".

Chapter XII

Stretching

Stretching is another important tool to promote physical, mental and emotional well-being.

Until the advent of the Industrial Revolution, our ancestors did not have problems resulting from a sedentary life. They had to work hard to satisfy the human being's most basic need: survival. As a result they stayed strong and healthy through continuous and energetic outdoor work.

From the energy point of view, physical exercise has the power not only of improving energy circulation but also grounding the individual. However, in a modern society where "pressing buttons" seems to be most people's main activity, it is not difficult to understand why we are dealing with so many physical and emotional problems.

Sedentary life => Energy stagnation => Mind & Body Disharmony

If one sees the world as being "grey", sitting in front a TV holding a remote control in one hand and a bag of potato chips in the other, certainly will not help the situation. Incidentally, one of the main treatments for depression is physical activity, which "amazingly" brings considerable well-being to the sufferer. He or she is literally sweating it out!

For someone who is not used to performing vigorous physical activity, it is not easy to all of a sudden start engaging in strenuous exercises. It is important to slowly adjust to a new lifestyle and the best bridge is Stretching.

Stretching exercises are important because they keep the muscles supple and prepared for movement, and help one to make the daily transition from inactivity to vigorous activity without undue strain. The slow and easy movement seen in Yoga exercises and taught by many sports instructors not only improve the body's condition but also prevent common injuries such as shin splints, Achilles tendinitis, and sore shoulders and elbows.

According to Bob Anderson, in his book *Stretching*, regular stretching can promote the following:

- reduce muscle tension and make the body feel more relaxed
- help coordination by allowing for freer and easier movement
- increase range of motion
- prevent injuries such as muscle strains
- make strenuous activities easier like running, skiing, tennis, etc
- develop body awareness. As we stretch various parts of the body, we focus on them and get in touch with them.
- promote circulation
- relax the mind and tunes up the body.

From Chinese medicine's point of view, stretching stimulates the energy flowing through the meridians, since they are located along the muscles. Moreover, most important acupuncture points are found in the joints. In order to perform its many and complex movements, a joint needs to be nurtured by blood and Chi; therefore, there is a considerable concentration of blood and Chi around the joints. On the other hand, this characteristic also makes the joint vulnerable to blockages, to stagnation. Thus, physical activity like stretching is very important to assure proper circulation and, by extension, good health.

Nature should be our main reference. Observe the animals, specially cats. They are always stretching their bodies, which makes them flexible and elegant.

The following stretching exercises are designed not to develop muscles but rather to assess the meridians' condition and to correct them. Again, since mind, body and emotions are connected, by working on the meridians we can certainly deal with emotional issues as well.

Lung and Large Intestine Meridians (When dealing with sadness, melancholy)

Streching position 1

- Stretch both arms upwards making a semi-circle. Feel the stretch for a moment; a warmth sensation is normally felt at the radial aspect of the arms.

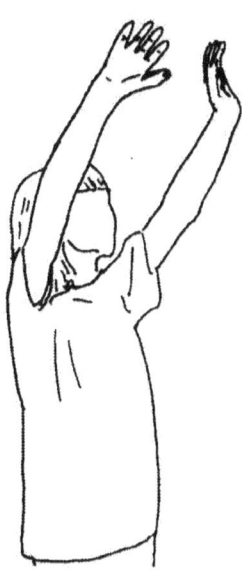

Fig. 1

Stretching position 2

- Clasp your hands behind your back. Bend forward and lift your arms as high as possible.

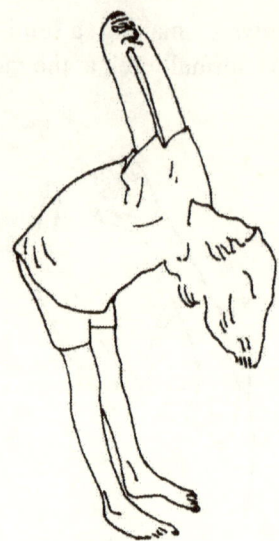

Fig. 2

Stomach and Spleen Meridians (When dealing with worry, preoccupation)

Stretching position 1
- Sit down with both legs bent (Japanese style) and lean straight backwards from that position, until your back lies flat on the floor.

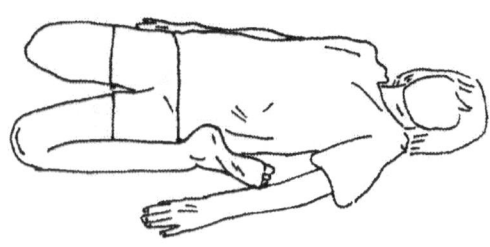

Fig. 3

Stretching position 2
- Alternatively, in case the first position feels too difficult to perform, one can just sit down with the left leg bent horizontal to the right first (feel the stretch); then do the same with the right leg.

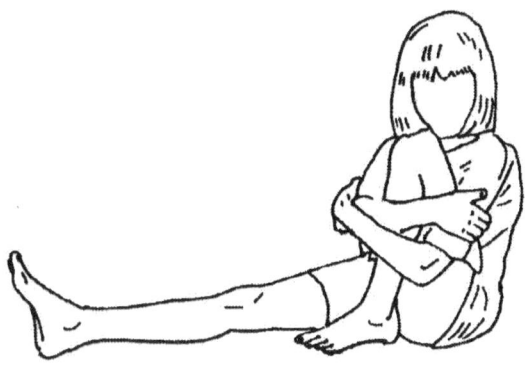

Fig. 4

Heart and Small Intestine Meridians (When dealing with bitterness, hysteria)

Stretching position 1
- Bring both arms behind you in a semi-circle; try bringing the little fingers close together. Hold the stretch for a while.

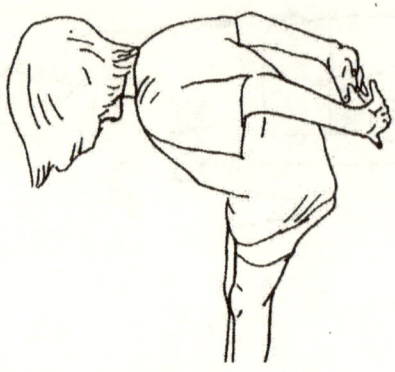

Fig. 5

Stretching position 2

- Bend one arm over your head (the arm can rest on the head), hold the stretch for a while, then do the same with the other arm.

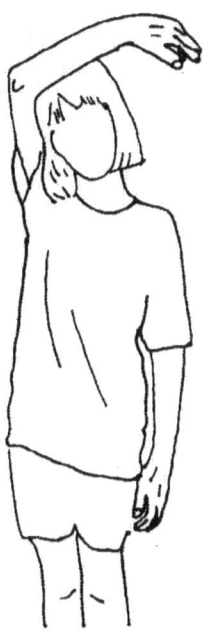

Fig. 6

Stretching position 3

- With the soles of your feet together, bring your feet towards your body as close as possible. Holding your feet with your hands, try touching your head to your toes resting your elbows on the floor. Relax as much as possible and take two deep breaths. If your knees don't lie flat on the floor, this indicates disharmony of the heart and small intestine meridians. This exercise helps to balance both meridians.

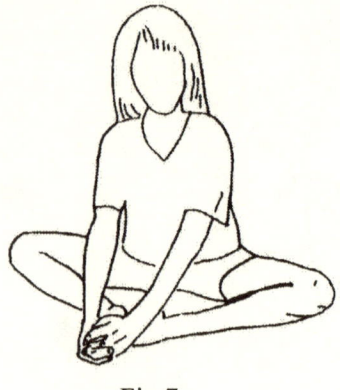

Fig.7

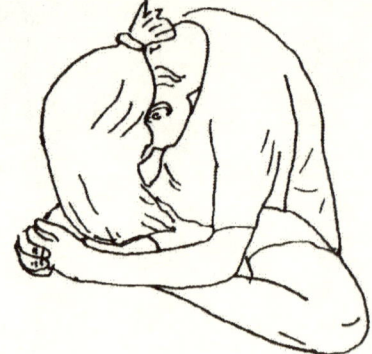

Fig.7.1

Kidney and Bladder Meridians (When dealing with fear, insecurity)

Stretching position 1

- Stretch your legs out in the front and touch your toes with your hands. Then bend forward and touch your head to your knees. At the maximum stretch point, relax completely and take two deep breaths. Any pain on one side indicates disharmony on the meridians on that side. This exercise harmonizes kidney and bladder meridians.

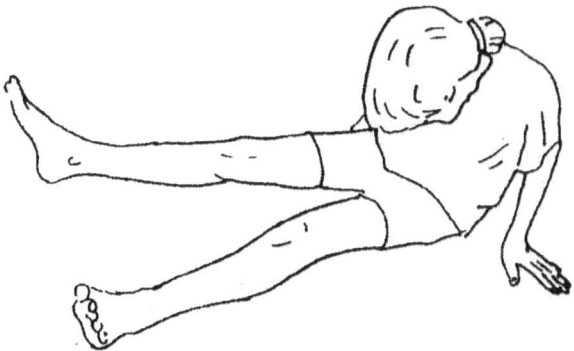

Fig. 8

Stretching position 2

- While lying down bend one leg with the sole touching the opposite hipbone. Hold the stretch for a moment, then do the same with the other leg. This will stimulate the bladder meridian.

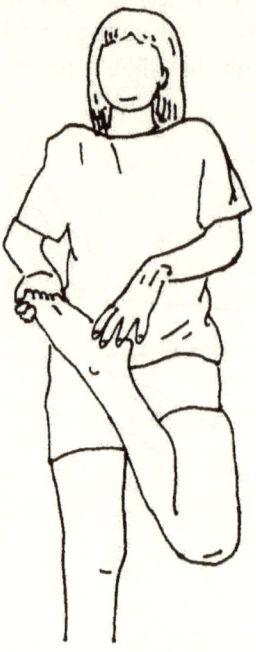

Fig.9

Stretching position 3

- While lying down, bend one knee and bring it close to your body. Hold it with both hands and feel the stretch for a while. This will stimulate the kidney meridian.

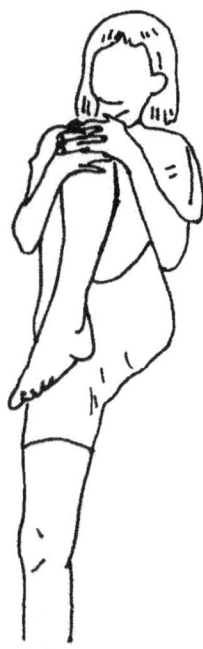

Fig.10

Liver and Gall Bladder Meridians (When dealing with anger, resentment, depression)

Stretching position 1

- Sitting with your legs spread as far as possible, touch your toes with the opposite hand. Do not bend your knees. At the maximum stretch point, take two deep breaths and relax completely. Any stiffness you may feel indicates disharmony of the meridians involved. This stretch harmonizes liver and gall bladder meridians.

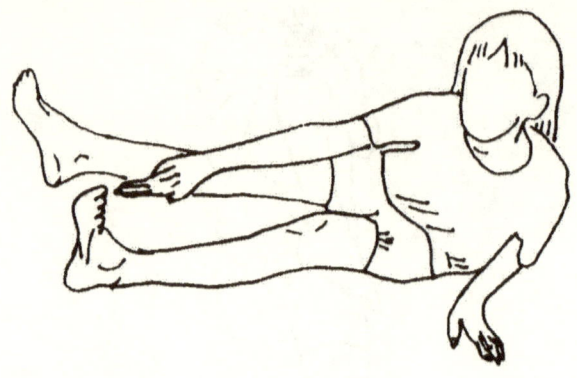

Fig.11

Stretching position 2

- While lying down, bend one leg with the sole of your foot touching the inside of the opposite knee, hold the stretch for a moment. Repeat the exercise with the other leg. This affects the liver meridian.

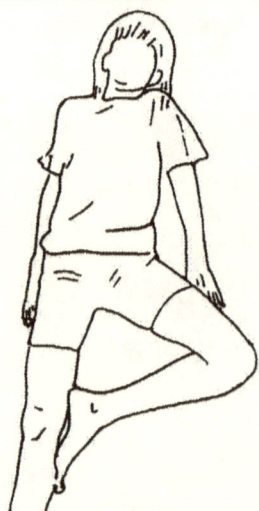

Fig.12

Stretching position 3

- While lying down, bend one knee with the sole of the foot lying flat on the floor. Lean the bent knee towards the opposite leg. Hold the stretch for a while. Repeat the exercise with the other leg. This stimulates the gall bladder meridian.

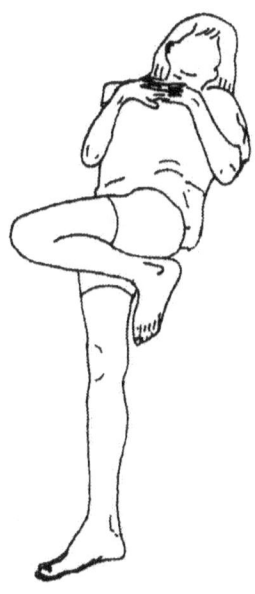

Fig.13

The above stretching exercises are recommended here for emotional problems, which are the object of this book. However, they certainly apply to all physical disharmony related to the meridians as well. They are useful and simple therapeutic tools. It is also important to say that stretching exercises are strongly recommended for everyone, whether experiencing a physiological or emotional symptom.

Chapter XIII

Breathing Techniques

There is a considerable variety of therapies, treatment styles and methods originated and/or developed in different parts of the world. However, there is a common element present in all of them: breathing. Yoga, Tai Chi Chuan, Qigong (Chi Kun), Holotropic Breathwork, and Relaxation Therapy are some of the techniques where breathing plays an important role.

Since breathing is coordinated by the autonomic nervous system, the system that controls our involuntary actions and reactions like breathing, hunger, sleeping, etc, we take it for granted; we are seldom aware of our breathing rhythms. However, professional and famous opera singers, musicians, athletes and actors know the importance of proper breathing in their performances. English Shakespearean actors know how crucial it is to develop breath control when performing.

Breathing is life. When we inhale we take not only oxygen into our lungs, but also vital energy that stimulates every single cell of our body. When we exhale, we get rid of not only physical toxins, but emotional ones as well. That is why traditional Oriental medicine stresses the importance of breathing exercises - to harmonize the body, mind and emotions. Breathing has a holistic effect.

Clinical studies prove that depending on our state of mind, brain waves can move at different frequencies. As we mentioned before, when we are mentally alert, thinking, worrying or anxious, the brain waves show a fast wave frequency (Beta Waves). In a more relaxed situation or meditative state, the frequency slows down considerably (Alpha Waves). Whereas, when one is in a deep meditative state or deep sleep the waves slow even more (Theta Waves), and so forth. However, the most important finding was that, through breathing exercises, *one could alter brain wave frequencies.*

Our body has mechanisms that stimulate the breathing frequency whenever we are engaged in strenuous physical activities, like jogging, doing aerobics, gymnastics or practising sports. On the other hand, our brain needs a considerable amount of oxygen in order to perform its functions properly; however, there is no special mechanism that stimulates our lungs to breathe more actively when we are thinking. Thus, whenever we are facing a challenge that requires mental work, we should pause once in a while and take some deep breaths; in so doing we may be able see things more clearly. So those persons whose jobs involve constant intellectual work should place a sign on their table which states: "Breathe; you are thinking!"

Chinese medicine considers breathing a force that propels Chi. It is so connected to our vital energy that many regard breath as being Chi itself. In fact, the energy that flows through our channel network is a combination of the pure essence extracted from the food we eat and the air we breathe. Through proper breathing, the Lungs send Chi down to the Kidneys, which return it back to the Lungs completing the "grand circulation". Whenever the Lungs or the Kidneys fail to perform that function or through inhaling toxic substances, like nicotine, the organs "lose contact" with each other and disease (specially respiratory problems) sets in.

As we have seen before, anxiety, sadness and emotions out of control can be harmonized through breathing exercises. Intentional and focused breathing can be an important therapeutic tool. Here are some examples:

Take a few minutes to yourself, find a comfortable position either sitting or preferably lying flat on the floor with arms relaxed by your side. Choose a breathing exercise that feels easy to you.

1 - *Staircase Breathing Exercise* — take a deep breath; hold it for a split second (feel the air inside your lungs) and breath out in "installments", slowly as if you were going down a staircase. Empty your lungs completely. Repeat the exercise for about ten times.

2 - *Counting Breaths Down to the Navel* - Take a slow and deep breath and exhale slowly, while visualizing the air being released all the way down to the navel. Repeat the exercise as many times as you feel comfortable.

3 - *Alternate Nostril Breathing* - This exercise is performed by using the right hand's thumb and ring finger. Close your right nostril with your right thumb and breathe out to the count of eight. Breathe in to the count of four and close your left nostril with the right ring finger. Hold for sixteen, then release your thumb and breathe out through the right nostril to the count of eight. Repeat the same exercise alternating the sides. This is a Yoga exercise normally performed in a sitting position. By alternating the breathing through left and right nostrils, both hemispheres of the brain are activated.

4 - *Breathing Exercise for Insomnia* - This exercise is best performed by lying down in a comfortable position, preferable in your bed ready to go to sleep. Place the left hand on the left hip bone and the right on top of the left hand. Breathe in while slowly sliding both hands up to the top of your chest (clavicle or collar bone); cross the chest and breathe out, while slowly sliding both hands down to your right hip bone. As you exhale, imagine that your hands are a steamroller that flattens your body getting rid of all stress, tension and anxiety. Do the exercise nine times, and before you know it you will be sound asleep.

Chapter XIV

Visualization Techniques

In my daily practice I have found Visualization to be a very effective therapy for stress and emotion-related problems. Quite often, regardless of the therapeutic line I choose to follow, I normally include it as part of the treatment with tangible results. The method is very simple and can be performed at home. In fact, I frequently prescribe the following visualization as a form of homework for my patients.

Firstly lie flat on the floor or bed with the arms by your side, as comfortably as possible. Close your eyes, take three deep breaths and imagine yourself inside your lungs. Now, visualize a pure white light surrounding and penetrating your *Lungs*. Be aware of any emotion, like sadness or melancholy. Visualize the emotions vanishing, disappearing in the presence of this *white* light. Feel your lungs rejuvenated and recharged with a powerful energy.

Next, imagine yourself inside your *Liver* at the right hand side under the ribcage. Now visualize a green light surrounding and penetrating your liver. Be aware of emotions like anger or resentment. Visualize those emotions fading away, vanishing in the presence of the *green* light. Feel your liver healthy and totally energized.

After that, imagine yourself back in the center of your chest, inside your *Heart*. Now, visualize a *red* light surrounding and penetrating your heart. Be aware of any emotions, like bitterness or restlessness. Visualize those feelings vanishing in the presence of the red light. Feel your heart strong, healthy and pacified.

Next, imagine yourself inside your *Stomach*. Now, visualize a *yellow* light surrounding and penetrating your stomach. Be aware of any tension or worrying. Visualize those sensations disappearing completely in the presence of the yellow light. Feel your digestive system strong and healthy.

After that, imagine yourself inside your *Kidneys*. Now, visualize a **dark blue** light surrounding and penetrating your kidneys. Be aware of emotions like fear and insecurity. Feel those emotions vanishing completely in the presence of the blue light. Experience a feeling of will power and strength taking over you.

Finally, visualize a ***purple*** cloud moving slowly from the top of your head to the tip of your toes. As it proceeds down your body, experience a profound relaxing sensation and harmony amongst all your organs.

Besides that, I usually recommend another powerful one for cases when there are relationship problems between husband and wife, siblings, parent and child or co-workers. I believe that most relationship problems result from two people vibrating at different frequencies. Thus, the following exercise helps two people to "communicate" with each other at the same frequency.

Find a quiet and comfortable spot. Sit down, close your eyes and take three nice deep breaths. Now, visualize the person you want your energy to harmonize with sitting in front of you. Try to picture the person as detailed as possible.

Ask that person (in your mind) what ***colour*** he/she needs from you. Pick the very first one that comes to your mind - no judgement! Now, imagine that colour coming from your chest, like a thick beam, and surrounding the person who is sitting in front of you. Let the colour bathe that person for a while.

Afterwards, when you think it is enough, imagine the person asking you what colour you need from him/her. Pick the first one that comes to your mind - again, no judgement! Visualize the colour emanating from his/her chest and bathing you for a while. Then, when the exercise is over, visualize the person surrounded by a pure white light and vanishing happily.

This exercise is very powerful and I have witnessed, as a therapist, many difficult cases of relationship problems being harmonized. However, it is common that in the beginning, the person who is doing the exercise cannot visualize anybody or any colour. Do not let that discourage you. Perseverance is the key to success.

I have an interesting case to report. A lady came to me for acupuncture treatment; she had a severe case of sciatica. As the treatment progressed, she complained that her real pain was caused by the lack of communication with her only son, who lived far away. The problem was that when her husband died, he left many failing businesses, and she had to sell part of their assets to settle all the debts. Her only son however, wouldn't forgive her for selling part of their holding and his consequently reduced inheritance. At that time it had been more than five years of silence, not a single letter or phone call.

Having heard that, I suggested she try the above exercise, which she put into practice immediately. After a short while of faithfully practising the visualization, her son, out of the blue, sent her a meaningful card and…to my amazement, the physical pain disappeared!

The ancient Chinese were aware of the power of the mind. In many old texts one can find expressions like "Where your mind is, your Chi is" and "Chi follows intention".

Therefore, one can use the power of positive thinking to bring about healing, not only of emotions but also of physical problems.

Chapter XV

Self-hypnosis

Every time I have to use the word *hypnosis*, when addressing the general public, I feel a bit uncomfortable. The main reason for this feeling lies in the fact that there are lots of misconceptions, mainly for those who have never experienced hypnotherapy. The idea of being helplessly "under somebody's powers" is perhaps the main one.

I have to confess that before studying hypnosis for therapy purposes, the only reference I had was stage hypnosis, where supposedly people were "told" to perform strange acts. In fact there is no such thing as giving up one's control. During a regular hypnotherapy session, the person is *totally* aware of what is going on; the hearing gets very sharp and the individual experiences nothing but a comfortable relaxation. He/she also allows himself/herself to be in that stage by choice, for all the client has to do is to open the eyes to terminate the session. In stage hypnosis the most susceptible people are chosen, but nobody can be forced to do something against his/her moral values. That is, however, a small aspect of hypnosis especially if we compare the enormous benefits it can offer when used as a therapeutic tool.

Generally speaking, we have two main levels of consciousness: the conscious and the subconscious mind. The conscious mind is the one that reflects, ponders and rationalizes. The subconscious mind does not analyze or judge any new information: *it just registers and stores it as true.* This is particularly common during our childhood, when our conscious mind is still immature and not capable of a sound judgement. When the child begins to be exposed to other children, at school, for instance, many bits of distorted information are stored in the subconscious mind.

"You have big ears" or "You have a monkey's face". These are examples of expressions that can be said to someone, who can discard them as a joke. However, a child not being mature enough to understand their real meaning of them, can take them seriously and the subconscious mind registers the information as real. Later on as an adult, the person may not recall the experience but the early input is there and can cause many problems.

In fact the hypnotherapy mechanism is very simple. By relaxing the body and the mind, the therapist can "bypass" the so-called *critical factor*, a normal conscious mind's reaction when given suggestions considered unrealistic, like "You are no longer a smoker" - to a heavy smoker, for instance. So, in a relaxed state, the subconscious mind can be accessed, any eventual "bad programs" erased and positive ones "planted". For those who find this far-fetched, remember the old cliché: We use only 10% of our brain's capacity!

Sometimes, instead of using the word *hypnosis* I employ the term *progressive relaxation*, because that is what the whole process is all about. In order to achieve good results, the therapist has to apply techniques that induce the subject to relax deeply. Again, with the body relaxed and the mind peaceful one can more effectively access the subconscious mind.

Another important feature of hypnosis is that a suggestion needs to be repetitive. That means, in order for the subconscious mind to erase the old program and to accept a new one, the latter needs to be vocalized repetitively. A good example of this is the strategy employed by TV advertising agencies. You hear a positive ad about a product over and over again (preferably associated with nice music, good health or success). The next time you go to a food store, before you know it, you are buying the product.

Quite recently there was an interesting experiment carried out by a school for mentally challenged children in the US. For a long time, there were many attempts to find the best method to teach the children to read with no major breakthrough. One day, however, one of the teachers noticed that the children were able to repeat many TV ads (words and songs included). With that information in mind the instructors began to use the TV ads' strategy: repetition with music in the background with considerable success.

Regular hypnotherapy sessions are advised for complex emotional problems or when the person feels impotent to help himself /herself. A good therapist has the experience to choose the best way to conduct the therapy that best suits the individual, according to the extension or magnitude of the problem. In normal circumstances, however, we are capable of trying to help ourselves to harmonize our emotions by using simple methods, like Self-Hypnosis.

As the name suggests, self-hypnosis is a technique that helps us to reach our subconscious mind through self-inducing a deep state of relaxation. The best way of doing this is by using a tape recorder. You can use a pre-recorded tape with instructions performed by a therapist or, even better, record your own. The main guidelines are:

1. The suggestions should be made as if somebody is talking to you, for instance: "Relax your body" or "Imagine that your legs are as light as feathers".

2. It is important to create messages that induce peace, relaxation and harmony. Sometimes quiet soothing music in the background helps tremendously.

3. If the purpose of the exercise is to deal with an emotional issue, avoid mentioning it because it would only emphasize its presence. Try choosing uplifting words; after all you are "planting" a positive program in your subconscious mind. Instead of saying, "You are no longer sad" say, "You are happy and cheerful."

4. Concentration is one of the keys to a successful session. Try concentrating on the voice, in this case, your recorded voice. Just say to yourself that any background noise would only deepen your relaxation even more.

5. Choose a very comfortable place and make sure that you will be undisturbed for as long as the session lasts. Lie down or if you fall easily asleep try sitting in a cozy chair, for it is important that despite being relaxed you can hear every word.

6. As we have seen before, breathing is very important. Therefore, before you begin, take long, deep and slow breaths; that will help you reach deeper levels of relaxation.

7. The relaxation should be induced by guided imagery, meaning "the voice" should guide your thoughts with words that create images to inspire relaxation. You can write well chosen words that apply to the case and read them in a soft and clear voice on the microphone moving slowly through the text and pausing often between sentences.

8. A good example of an induction text is the one that focuses on relaxing each part of your body, either beginning from your head or your toes. I find that moving up is more effective, since it creates a certain expectation. So here is a common pattern:

Now that your are comfortably lying down (or sitting), take some long and deep breaths. As you breath in and breathe out, be aware of the importance of respiration. During this process, your body brings in not only air, but also fresh and cooling energy that stimulates your lungs and every single cell of your body. As you breathe out, your body gets rid of physical, mental and emotional toxins as well.

As you get more comfortable, I would like you to divert your attention to your right foot. Relax your right foot. Relax your toes, your tendons and ankles. Just imagine that your right foot is a rag-doll; no tension whatsoever.

Now, just pretend that a wave of relaxation is moving up your right leg. Feel your calf totally relaxed. As the wave moves up, relax your right knee; all around it; outside, inside, back and front. Then feel this relaxation moving from your knee all the way up to your hipbone. Your right leg is totally and completely relaxed.

Now, I would like you to shift your attention to your left foot. Relax your left foot; the tendons and the ankles. Feel this wave of relaxation moving up to your left calf, your left knee, all the way to your left hipbone. Both of your legs are totally and completely relaxed. They feel like feathers: no weight whatsoever.

The wave of relaxation now moves to your abdomen. Relax the area around your navel. If there is any tension in that area, make it disappear. Next, relax your chest. Be aware of any stress or tension that might be in your chest, as you breathe. Make it fade away and allow a deep sensation of peace and harmony to take over.

Now relax your shoulders, your arms, elbows, wrists, hands and fingers. Just feel both arms very light with no tension whatsoever.

Feel the waves of relaxation moving up to your neck - all around: the back, front and sides of your neck. Make all the tension disappear. Relax your mouth, all the muscles around your mouth. Relax your ears, your nose, your eyes, the muscles around your eyes and the forehead. Feel this amazing sense of well being and relaxation taking over your entire body, from the top of your head to the tip of your toes.

At this point your should be very relaxed but there is also a technique to deepen the feeling even more:

Now that your body and your mind are completely relaxed, lets go to deeper levels of relaxation. Imagine that you are on top of a staircase. The staircase has ten steps. As we go down the steps, you will be experiencing a gradual deepening of the relaxation you now have. So, ten…nine…eight…seven…six…five…four… three…two …one. Now, imagine that you are lying down on a feather mattress. Your body is light and your mind at peace.

Now your subconscious mind is open to suggestions. You can record any message you find useful to heal the emotional wound. Try choosing specific words that serve as an "antidote" to the problem. Again, try to speak slowly, clearly and most importantly, repeat the message for at least three times.

Examples:

When dealing with sadness: *Breathe in and breathe out. As you breathe in, feel the joy, this wonderful and nurturing feeling entering your chest and spreading throughout your entire body. Every single cell is sparkling with joy, bliss and ecstasy.*

When dealing with fear: *Feel this powerful wave of warm energy taking over your body, beginning from your feet and moving up, taking over your entire body. You are a child of the Creator. It took tremendous energy for nature to create you, to give you life. Likewise, you have the power to create your own destiny.*

When dealing with anger: *Your body is so light that it feels like a feather, which is blown by the wind gently swings down to the ground. Harmony surrounds you and takes over your whole being. Your heart is at peace.*

When dealing with worry: *As you breathe in and breathe out, your mind is at peace and your body experiences a deep feeling of relaxation. Everything is* fine and all is well. Trust the Universe, your path, your mind, your body and your soul.

When dealing with depression: *The more you relax, the more your cells rejuvenate and energize. All functions of your body are activated: your mind is alert, your blood circulation is improved, the energy flows easily. You are experiencing a powerful sensation taking over your whole being. Life is movement and you are perfectly in tune with it. You are in control.*

When dealing with guilt: *You are a dear child of the Universe. Your journey is beginning now. The experiences of the past help you pave your new way - you are more mature, experienced and wise. Forgive everyone, all the past experiences, forgive yourself; you are free. Repeat the last sentence three times in the first person: I forgive...I am free!*

The suggestions above are just examples of the messages you want to "implant" in your subconscious mind. You can create, expand and mold them to your own needs. The more you repeat them, the more chances you have of being successful. It is important to remember:

Relaxed body + relaxed mind → access to subconscious mind

Closing Words From The Author

Knowledge is a road with no U-turns. Every time we learn something new, like a new language, information or skill, our brain cells take a different configuration and expand. We can call this "expansion of the mind".

The material presented in this work aims to expand your awareness about the effects of the emotions on the body. It is my wish that these simple yet profound ideas, known to the Chinese 5000 years ago, resonate deeply within you and that you can apply them in your daily lives. Only by understanding the energy link between the mind and the body are we able to identify patterns of disharmony before they manifest themselves as diseases.

There is an old Chinese saying that can be translated as, "Only when we unite our mind to our heart will we attain enlightenment." This can be the first step.

I wish you peace and harmony in all aspects of your life.

Cairo P Rocha

Bibliography

XINNONG, Cheng. *Chinese Acupuncture and Moxibustion.* Beijing, China: Foreign Language Press, 1987.

MACIOCIA, Giovanni. *The Foundations of Chinese Medicine.* UK: Churchill Livingstone, 1989.

ELMAN, Dave. *Hypnotherapy.* Glendale, CA: Westwood Publishing Co., 1964.

PITCHFORD, Paul. *Healing with Whole Foods: Oriental Traditions and Modern Nutrition.* Berkeley, CA: North Atlantic Books, 1993.

LARRE, Claude and Elisabeth Rochat de la Vallee. *The Seven Emotions. Psychology and Health in Ancient China.* Cambridge, UK: Monkey Press, 1996.

GIMBEL, Theo. *Healing Through Colours.* Essex, UK: C.W.Daniel, 1980.

GIMBEL, Theo. *Form, Sound, Colour and Healing.* Essex, UK: C.W.Daniel, 1987.

BARNARD, Julian. *A Guide to Bach Flower Remedies.* Essex, UK: C.W.Daniel, 1987

TOO, Lillian. *Applied Pa-Kua and Lo Shu Feng Shui.* Adelaide, Australia: Oriental Publications, 1993.

TSE, Michael. *Qi Magazine.* Manchester, UK: Tse Qigong Centre, Issue 31, 1997.

MORIN, John. *The Ultimate Origuml Book.* Philadelphia, Pennsylvania: Courage Books, 1998.

ANDERSON, Bob. *Stretching.* Bolinas, California: Shelter Publications, Inc., 1980.

COOPER, J.C. *Chinese Alchemy: The Taoist Quest for Immortality.* N.Y.: Sterling Publishing Co., Inc., 1990.

MATSUNAGA, Shizuto and Wataru Ohashi. *Zen Shiatsu.* Tokyo: Japan Publications, Inc., 1977.

About the Author

Since 1983 Cairo Rocha has been teaching and practicing acupuncture. After receiving a law degree from the University of Brasilia, Brazil, he traveled to Tokyo, Japan where he completed a four-year degree in Oriental Medicine. He studied co-related natural therapies in Germany, France and Scotland and has since been practicing in Brasilia and, more recently, in Nassau, Bahamas .Cairo has recently integrated hypnotherapy into his practice and has given workshops on various aspects of Chinese medicine throughout Brazil, the Bahamas, the United States and the UK.

For information about workshops and seminars visit: www.cairorocha.com

www.ingramcontent.com/pod-product-compliance
Lightning Source LLC
Chambersburg PA
CBHW051437280526
45785CB00003B/1322